CHRONIC PAIN AND BRAIN ABNORMALITIES

CHRONIC PAIN AND BRAIN ABNORMALITIES

Editor

CARL Y. SAAB

Brown University, Providence, RI, USA

AMSTERDAM • BOSTON • HEIDELBERG • LONDON
NEW YORK • OXFORD • PARIS • SAN DIEGO
SAN FRANCISCO • SINGAPORE • SYDNEY • TOKYO

Academic Press is an imprint of Elsevier

Academic Press is an imprint of Elsevier
32 Jamestown Road, London NW1 7BY, UK
225 Wyman Street, Waltham, MA 02451, USA
525 B Street, Suite 1800, San Diego, CA 92101-4495, USA

British Library Cataloguing-in-Publication Data
A catalogue record for this book is available from the British Library

Library of Congress Cataloging-in-Publication Data
A catalog record for this book is available from the Library of Congress

ISBN: 978-0-12-398389-3

For information on all Academic Press publications
visit our website at elsevierdirect.com

Typeset by MPS Limited, Chennai, India
www.adi-mps.com

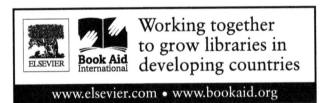

Working together
to grow libraries in
developing countries

www.elsevier.com • www.bookaid.org

Dedication

To Rafa, Sofia and Adam who promised to read this book, one day

Short Contents

Full Contents

Preface

This book is largely the brainchild of conversations ad-hoc to the Society for Neuroscience annual convention in Washington D.C., November 2011. I had the honor and privilege at that event to chair a Symposium entitled "Chronic Pain and Brain Abnormalities" by leading experts in the field of pain physiology. The speakers, including several of the authors of this book, discussed clinical data showing electrophysiological evidence for aberrant neural activity in the brains of patients with chronic pain, in parallel with basic science evidence from animal models of pain, which was corroborated by imaging data suggestive of disrupted brain networks. Soon after the symposium, it became clear that the subject matter and the topics presented merited follow-up discussions in a book format. Such a book, we hoped, would offer the reader better appreciation of the fundamentals of pain-related abnormalities in the brain, as well as present and futuristic overviews of emerging neurotechnological and theoretical tools available to study these changes.

When John Lorber was presented with a young student of an above average IQ, a first-class honors degree in mathematics, and normal social skills, yet had virtually 'no brain' due to severe hydrocephalus, he asked rhetorically "is a brain really necessary?".[1] Dr. Lorber further contended "there must be a tremendous amount of redundancy or spare capacity in the brain, just as there is with kidney and liver." Indeed, a skeptic may question whether a brain is at all necessary for pain, and if so, which parts of it? Our response is that great strides have been made recently that have helped us better tackle such dramatic claims by showing that not only is a brain obviously necessary for the pain experience, but that a brain needs to function properly within a very narrow range of activity patterns to allow for normal feelings and thought processes. Disrupting the exact timing of action potential discharges of single neurons within a millisecond range, or shifting network oscillations between neuronal networks by a few Hz may lead to devastating effects at the sensory and cognitive levels.

We believe this book provides broad scholarly references for pain practitioners, clinicians, scientists, therapists and biomedical engineers inspiring to design the next generation neurotechnologies for probing brain circuitry and modulating brain function. We share the vision that research into the mechanisms of pain in the brain, whether considered simply correlative to, or causative of the pain experience, is a win–win strategy that will potentially bring chronic pain patients closer to objective diagnostics and more effective therapies.

Carl Y. Saab, Editor

Reference

1. Lewin R. Is your brain really necessary? *Science.* 1980;210(4475):1232–1234.

List of Contributors

Daniel M. Aghion   Department of Neurosurgery, Rhode Island Hospital and Hasbro Children's Hospital and Brown University, Alpert School of Medicine, Providence, RI, USA

Radi Al-Masri   Department of Endodontics, Prosthodontics and Operative Dentistry, Baltimore College of Dental Surgery, University of Maryland Baltimore, Baltimore, MD, USA

Lino Becerra   P.A.I.N. Group, Boston Children's Hospital, Harvard Medical School, Waltham, MA, USA

David Borsook   P.A.I.N. Group, Boston Children's Hospital, Harvard Medical School, Waltham, MA, USA

Garth Rees Cosgrove   Department of Neurosurgery Rhode Island Hospital and Hasbro Children's Hospital and Brown University, Alpert School of Medicine, Providence, RI, USA

Asaf Keller   Department of Anatomy and Neurobiology, University of Maryland School of Medicine, Baltimore, MD, USA

J.H. Kim   Department of Neurosurgery, Ansan Hospital, Korea University, Seoul, Korea

K. Kobayashi   Department of Neurological Surgery, Division of Applied Systems Neuroscience, and Department of Advanced Medical Science, Nihon University, Tokyo, Japan

Frederick A. Lenz   Department of Neurosurgery, Johns Hopkins University, Baltimore, MD, USA

C.C. Liu   Department of Neurosurgery, Johns Hopkins University, Baltimore, MD, USA

Rodolfo R. Llinás   Department of Physiology & Neuroscience, NYU School of Medicine, New York, NY, USA

T.M. Markman   Department of Neurosurgery, Johns Hopkins University, Baltimore, MD, USA

Eric Moulton   P.A.I.N. Group, Boston Children's Hospital, Harvard Medical School, Waltham, MA, USA

Eric Newman   P.A.I.N. Group, Boston Children's Hospital, Harvard Medical School, Waltham, MA, USA

Carl Y. Saab   Brown University, Providence, RI, USA

Kerry Walton   Department of Physiology & Neuroscience, NYU School of Medicine, New York, NY, USA

J.C. Zhang   Department of Neurosurgery, Johns Hopkins University, Baltimore, MD, USA

List of Figures

1

Introduction

Carl Y. Saab

Brown University, Providence, RI, USA

"We are all bitched from the start and you especially have to be hurt like hell before you can write seriously. But when you get the damned hurt use it—don't cheat with it. Be as faithful to it as a scientist." **Ernest Hemingway to F. Scott Fitzgerald.**

"Pain is the question mark turned like a fishhook in the human heart." **Peter De Vries.**

RATIONALE AND SCOPE OF THIS BOOK

This book focuses on the neurophysiological mechanisms of pain in the brain, in particular chronic pain conditions. Chronic pain is broadly defined as a myriad of long-lasting, poignantly unpleasant sensations, in addition to a host of cognitive, behavioral and emotional comorbidities that are not alleviated by standard pharmacotherapy. It is a state of consciousness that deviates from common painful experiences in ways that profoundly threaten the patient's wellbeing and quality of life. A more elaborate definition of chronic pain is discussed below, and the authors have each attempted to articulate the specific chronic pain condition in question, as there are many that manifest with different etiologies, symptomatology and, arguably, physiological mechanisms.

Certain forms of chronic pain such as neuropathic pain, are classified as neurological disorders, begging the question "where in the nervous system is the pathology?" Can one speak of pathogenesis and etiology of chronic pain in classical terms such as the pathogenesis of cancer or the etiology of cystic fibrosis? Restricted lesions in the brain have been known to lead to central pain, for example thalamic pain syndrome due to a stroke in the thalamus. However, the authors of this book do not wish to generalize that the brain is the target organ of pathology in patients suffering from all sorts of chronic pain, the same way for example that joint pathology is the ubiquitous cause for arthritis. Rather, we endorse the view that brain mechanisms associated with chronic pain could provide valuable clues to the underlying neural circuitry that is *required* for the pain experience. This perspective should not be construed as pointing fingers at "pain centers" in the brain that set off a host of feelings and emotions intimately entwined with pain.

Accordingly, my main goal as Editor was to engage leading clinicians and scientists in the pain field to reconcile the wealth of clinical and laboratory data in one book, to place these data within a coherent hypothetical framework, and to discuss up-to-date therapeutic options that target the brain exclusively. In my opinion, the authors have done an excellent job in identifying a set of measurable neurophysiological phenomena that are highly correlated with the pain experience (i.e. predictive of pain), and phenomena whose modulation could alter the pain experience (i.e. of potential therapeutic value).

With these disclaimers in mind, it would be presumptuous (even nonsensical) to claim that, one day, given the right technology, we'll be able to visualize what pain looks like in the brain. What we are prepared to say, instead, is that we are now closer to predicting pain in others with a high degree of confidence based on empirical measures. Moreover, we hope that similar approaches might, at the very least, help guide future diagnostics, and also, in the best case scenario, inform novel therapies.

WHAT IS PAIN?

Can pain be accurately defined? Several authoritative books on pain have only partially succeeded in defining the pain experience in a fully comprehensive manner.[1–7] Even one of the most widely-used definitions of pain among medical and academic professionals (which was formulated by the International Association for the Study of Pain, IASP[8]) falls short of grasping the pain experience in its entirety from the genealogy, etiology, epistemology and phenomenology perspectives* (see below). It is not surprising that linguists and philosophers across ages have been fascinated with the human experience of pain as a subject of study. Unless the reader is born with a genetic predisposition for pain insensitivity,[9] they will unequivocally understand what pain means without further elaboration. This concept of perfectly understanding (or relating to) a phenomenon, yet not being able to reach universal agreement over its definition using communicable language, is not unique to pain.

---

*"Pain is an unpleasant sensory and emotional experience associated with actual or potential tissue damage or described in terms of such damage." "Many people report pain in the absence of tissue damage or any likely pathophysiological cause; usually this happens for psychological reasons."

Consider for example the word "game." Try as you may to reach a consensus on a definition of what game is (or what it is *not*), even among your closest friends, game will still mean different things to different people. Yet, call on someone to "play a game," the person would likely engage in that specific activity (knowing the rules governing that game) without invoking a philosophical conundrum. It is argued that terms such as "game," "love" and "pain" are understood because of community agreement about what these terms refer to, irrespective of our inability to confine them within the boundaries of common language. Therefore they are said to be representations of knowledge only partially anchored in language, and can only be conveyed most sincerely and gracefully by "showing" rather than by "saying": "There are, indeed, things that cannot be put into words. They *make themselves manifest*. They are what is mystical"[10] (p. 89); "What we cannot speak about we must pass over in silence"[10](p. 89*). This is why, it is assumed, when two individuals communicate their pain experiences to one another, they can be said to play a language game whose rules follow popular votes far from being rigid (see "Private Language and Rule-Following Arguments").[11] Accordingly, one expects the qualifiers of the human pain experience to change dramatically with time and across cultures. Indeed, chilling accounts of pain insensitivity based on race portray a disturbing cultural bias and a racial rapport to pain ("Negresses will bear cutting with nearly, if not quite, as much impunity as dogs and rabbits"[5], p. 40). Furthermore, the rising epidemic of pain hints at a possible shift in the collective pain barometer in modern days. Compare our daily moaning and groaning about back pain and joint pain with anecdotal accounts of Greek and Trojan wartime injuries, which are described with anatomical precision in *The Iliad*, however, with no hint of suffering or agony that live up to the traumatic atrocities they endured.[5] It seems that the boundary of language cowers to pain, and one is inclined, thereof, to accept Wittgenstein's position, that the genuine definition of a word lies in its use ("Don't Think but Look!" *aphorism 66*[12]).

---

*Tractatus Logico-Philosophicus is the only philosophical work published by Ludwig Wittgenstein during his lifetime (1889–1951), with an introduction by his mentor Bertrand Russel. It was first published in *Annalen der Naturphilosophie* in 1921, followed by the English translation in 1922. It is written in short, hierarchically numbered statements with seven basic propositions at the primary level (1–7) and sub-level statements at decimal places thereof, portraying extreme compression and brilliance. The quotations here refer to original statements numbered 6.522 and 7, respectively. Wittgenstein became very critical of his own work soon after publication. More of his work resurfaced posthumously, including *Philosophical Investigations*, also written in numbered paragraphs referred to as *aphorisms*.

PAIN IN ANIMALS

The difficulty in communicating one's own pain experience is even more compounded when trying to appreciate someone else's pain, or pain in other species. However, after years of working with animal models of pain, there is no doubt in my mind that animals feel pain and suffer from it. With the absence of an algesiometer with which one could measure pain quantitatively and empirically, confirmation of pain in others (be it human, rat or fish) remains completely subjective and arbitrary. Perhaps the Wittgensteinian dictum "What we cannot speak about we must pass over in silence" applies aptly in the case of animals, whereby pain-like behavior is our best (or at least most reliable) indicator of their general state of physical suffering, for even "if a lion could speak, we wouldn't understand him"[12]*aphorism 223*). What's left for an observer looking for clues about the sensory and emotional states of the wounded animal is a set of typical behaviors the observer can relate to, such as guarding the affected limb, vocalization, or alienation from its social milieu. However, the overwhelming majority of laboratory pain tests are based on so-called evoked responses to noxious stimuli, which involve recording the time it takes for an injured animal to withdraw the affected limb being stimulated with a moderately noxious heat stimulus, or in response to a moderately noxious mechanical stimulus. Some advances in the development of novel testing paradigms, such as place preference[13] and coding of facial grimaces,[14] have offered interesting alternatives to the traditional withdrawal reflex-based behavior. These inherent pitfalls associated with the use of behavior (reflexive and/or operant) as surrogate for predicting pain in animals have served as the platform for mounting serious criticism against the translational value of animal models. Regardless, pre-clinical animal models of pain have played—and continue to play—a key role in basic laboratory pain research.

PAIN WE NEED

Evading hurt and suffering, or quickly eliminating either when they happen, is a guiding principle for many of us. Avoiding pain and discomfort may be the single most important factor influencing our day-to-day decisions, whereby "the right to a pain-free life" has attained an almost human right status. However, one must not confuse this tenet with striving to be pain-insensitive. This nuance is critical for the understanding of the value of pain, which serves primarily as a protective function that's essential for survival. It is one thing to plan ahead to try to dodge as many painful stimuli as possible, and quite another to go through life without fear of harmful events, not knowing what pain is or what it means. For example, the fear of bee stings might prohibit a pain-sensitive person from reaching for honey from a beehive without the protective gear, whereas a pain-insensitive person with disregard for the bees warning signals might rush to the beehive with bare hands; the punishing experience of pain is just not there. In fact, congenital insensitivity to pain (CIP), a form of the rare hereditary sensory and autonomic neuropathies, is characterized from birth with a host of sensory deficits including mainly loss of pain and temperature (heat/cold) sensations, sleep disturbance and mental retardation (thought to be the result of the inability for thermoregulation during childhood in the case of CIP with anhydrosis).[9] Though not directly fatal, the life expectancy of people with CIP is less than 25 years, which is mainly attributed to unattended severe traumatic injuries or infections. Other clinical conditions associated with partial pain insensitivity in the distal limbs include leprosy, leading to tissue wasting and amputation. Interestingly, the challenge for leprosy patients presenting with distal neuropathy is restoring their ability to feel pain in the affected limbs, or at least train them to better protect and safeguard their limbs, which has proven to be a difficult, if not impossible, task.[15] In fact, Paul Brand, a pioneer in leprosy treatment, went on to develop a "prosthetic pain system," using mechanical sensors in gloves and socks that deliver electric shock to a sensitive part of the body (armpit). However, Dr. Brand relinquished his pursuit saying:

> In the end we had to abandon the entire scheme. Most important, we found no way around the fundamental weakness in our system: it remained under the patient's control. If the patient did not want to heed the warnings from our sensory [prosthetic], he could always find a way to bypass the whole system. Why must pain be unpleasant? Why must pain persist? Our system failed for the precise reason that we could not effectively duplicate those two qualities of pain. *Brand*[16] *(p. 195).*

Nevertheless, he continued to expand on the techniques for protecting the insensitive foot and hand in novel ways, noting that:

> Pain is the most valuable sensation we have. Never minimize its value. Never suppress pain unless you know its cause and have dealt with the root of the problem. Work with the sensations of pain, not against them. Pain is the way your own cells talk to you; listen and obey. When you value your own sensations, give special care to those who suffer from having no pain.

One wonders whether the paraphernalia of current over-the-counter pain medication might be, in some way, counteracting our natural pain system and helping us sustain unhealthy behaviors by ignoring warning signals such as headache and joint pain.

PAIN WE DON'T NEED

Having argued that pain is a blessing, it must be said that this is mostly true in the case of normal pain. But is there such a thing as abnormal pain? As the total absence of pain can be detrimental to the few hundred documented cases of CIP, awkward and/or exaggerated and long-lasting pain seriously threatens the wellbeing of millions around the world. When the degree and quality of pain are uncoupled from apparent bodily injury, and if this pain persists for more than six months, is described in vague or unusual terms such as "electric-like" and/or evoked by gentle touch, it is mostly referred to as pathological chronic pain. Perhaps the best description of chronic pain comes from personal accounts of patients suffering from unremitting pain.

REAL FACES OF PAIN: CASE ILLUSTRATIONS

As discussed earlier regarding the difficulty of defining the word pain, and the highly idiosyncratic nature of chronic pain, it is helpful perhaps to use vivid illustrations of what chronic pain ought to look like in human subjects, thereby portraying a certain profile of the common chronic pain patient. Indeed, providing intimate descriptions of real case studies is important in going beyond the strict clinical jargon of medical charts and straight into the core issues of the pain patient's feelings. Profound feelings of helplessness and anxiety (more so than depression), sadness, and a general sense of grief or loss tend to be common among those that experience severe pain that goes unabated for more than a straight three or six months period (p. 33). To a busy clinician, this added "baggage of feelings" amounts to nothing but a nuisance and a waste of time during consultation, whereas to an astute pain specialist they represent valuable signs that reinforce the medical diagnosis and, in some cases, mitigate suspicions of malingering (an important medico-legal issue beyond the scope of this book, p. 9).

Other common denominators of the chronic pain patient include a set of social or behavioral attributes such as difficulty in coping with daily activities, heavy use of heath care services (often in a futile quest of finding an elusive "cure"), as well as clear evidence of hightened psychological disturbances (though not necessarily psychiatric illnesses *per se*). In brief, reciprocal interactions between the patient and their social networks considered immediate (for example family members) and intermediate (neighbors, co-workers) become severely strained. Here again, it is the job of the health care provider to pick up the threads of these "emotional signs" that are interwoven with the "biological symptoms" (for example in the case of cancer pain) to reach a definitive diagnosis and start the patient on a course of effective pain management, which, in an ideal setting, requires a multidisciplinary approach.

Two case histories are described below, based on personal observations (Ms. A) and as reported by Ranjan Roy (Mr. B,[17]):

Ms. A incurred avulsion fracture to ankle at the age of 12. Soon after, she developed sensitivity to touch, burning pain, and cold up to her knee, along with bluish coloration in the extremities and extreme pain upon application of ice on the discolored body parts. She was diagnosed with chronic pain secondary to reflex sympathetic dystrophy (RSD) by her first physician (Dr. 1) within three weeks after initial injury. She immediately began physical therapy but her symptoms did not improve. She underwent lumbar sympathetic block by Dr. 2, but her symptoms did not improve either. Confused but willing to pursue non-traditional therapies, she moved to another state and was treated by Dr. 3 with two regional intravenous blocks and physical therapy. She returned to her home state the following year and continued with physical therapy, acupuncture, and biofeedback. However, she later stopped acupuncture due to pain spreading to her left hand and arm, but began walking roughly one year after her initial ankle injury. Meanwhile, she continued to "try" different medications including, but not limited to: Norco, Neurontin, Nortriptyline, Lamical, Clonidine, Fentanyl patches, Celebrex, Oxycontin, and Lyrica. Six years after initial injury, a spinal cord stimulator was implanted on her left side, with RSD spreading to her left leg with occasional full body flare-ups. Eight years on, with pain unabated, she decided to stop all medications and the spinal cord stimulator was removed eleven years after initial injury. Twelve years after initial injury, she underwent minor surgery for a fifth metatersal osteotomy in the left foot, which unfortunately caused a severe RSD flare up. At the last check, she was considering Low Dose Naltrexone and minocycline. Her pain, more than a decade after being diagnosed with RSD, can be described as deep bone pain, prickles, vibration sensation, cold limbs, occasional burning and sensitivity to touch, accompanied by muscle twitches and color change. In spite of her condition, she enjoys Pilates and stationary cycling.

Framed within a social context, Ranjan Roy's interesting interpretation of the detailed history of a pain patient portrays a man's concealed plight for help in dealing with stressful life events under the guise of severe headaches[17] (p. 31).

> Mr. B, at age 69 presented with a prolonged history of head pain which had worsened some three years ago at the time of his retirement. The curious aspect of his case was that despite the long history of pain, Mr. B had never sought professional help until his retirement. Even then he refused to take medication for pain. Generally, he was in excellent health. Mr. B had retired as a vice-president of a multinational firm, but he continued to pursue his numerous charitable and community

activities. Mr. B, during the first interview at the pain clinic, showed very little interest in discussing his headaches. Rather, he reflected on his wife's diabetes, which has led to her blindness. He spoke without emotion, almost with clinical detachment. He was not prone to being emotional, and no one could accuse him of losing his temper. The communicative significance of Mr. B's headaches as a mode of expressing distress was unmistakable. Expression of negative emotions was not in his repertoire. Conflicts had to be avoided at any cost. His indifference to his headaches raised the question of his real reasons for seeking help. For a man of his intellect and personality, seeking help through physical symptoms was more acceptable. His overwhelming feelings of anger, loss, and sadness were revealed only in the course of psychotherapy.

Several features of these testimonials are unfortunately common to many chronic pain patients, such as inaccurate early on diagnosis and a host of co-morbid conditions including depression, loss of appetite, lack of sleep and weight loss, leading to job loss, social alienation, dependency, and in some severe cases suicide.[18] It is thought that the typical chronic pain patient will experience on average 4–5 referrals before reaching a satisfactory diagnosis, and that some clinicians would consider pain medication to be effective if it barely leads to 25–50% pain reduction in just about 50% of patients. A detailed discussion of the different types of chronic pain and their etiologies would take up an entire monogram. Instead, the reader is referred to other well-written references on this topic.[19,20]

PAIN; MORE THAN A NUMBERS GAME

Knowledge about the prevalence of chronic pain in society and its associated health care costs helps in appreciating the magnitude and scale of this condition, compared with other types of medical conditions, especially for policy makers and funding agencies. Though an accurate prediction of the number of individuals with chronic pain has been elusive, there is little if any disagreement that chronic pain reached endemic proportions both nationally and globally. Latham and Davis[21] estimated that chronic pain is the third largest healthcare problem in the world, afflicting approximately 30% of the population globally.

Irrespective of sampling and other statistical discrepancies, the diagnostic criteria for chronic pain remain somewhat murky. Moreover, confirmation of pain conditions in the pediatric population and in patients with co-morbid psychiatric illnesses further limits the power of estimation of chronic pain in the population at large. Notwithstanding, the widely-cited Nurpin Pain Report,[22] based on a nationwide telephone survey, appears to provide reasonable quantitative data on the prevalence and severity of different kinds of pain in individuals aged 18 and older, representing a cross-section of the adult population in the United States.

The survey also claims to take into account the demographic characteristics of those with pain symptoms and the impact of pain on work and productivity. Interestingly, the report, published in 1986, concludes that 76.5 million individuals suffered from chronic pain, which, assuming a national census of approximately 233 million during that same year, amounts to a staggering 32% of the entire Unites States' population. Interestingly, a recent report by the Institute of Medicine of the National Academies provides an updated approximation closer to 100 million Americans, which perfectly matches with the 32% prevalence 25 years earlier (assuming a current census of 313 million Americans in 2012). By way of comparison, a recent study characterized the persistence of pain in the general population in Norway, while aiming to validate recall measures against longitudinal reporting of pain at 12-month follow-up.[23] Based on a random sample of more than 6000 participants (the HUNT 3 study in Norway), the calculated prevalence of chronic pain, classified as moderate or more, reached 26%. Though other studies have shown widely variable prevalence estimates of chronic pain ranging from 11% to 64%, thus creating uncertainty about the real extent of the problem, nearly all studies have concluded it is a major health issue, affecting more Americans than diabetes, heart disease and cancer combined*. With regards to expenses, health care bills associated with the diagnosis and treatment of chronic pain sum up to $6,280 per person annually. Consequently, the total costs of chronic pain are estimated at $600 billion. Compare that to high blood pressure, for example, which is prevalent at 40% globally but can reasonably be kept under control with typically less than $1,000 per person annually.

WHY FOCUS ON THE BRAIN? A PHILOSOPHICAL PERSPECTIVE

"We don't even know whether we are asking the right questions" *Nikola Grahek,*[4] *pxi.*

It is unavoidable here to invoke the most widely used definition by the IASP of pain as "an unpleasant sensory and emotional experience associated with actual or potential tissue damage or described in terms of such damage." The definition actually emphasizes that "many people report pain in the absence of tissue damage or any likely pathophysiological cause; usually this happens for psychological reasons. This definition avoids tying pain to the stimulus." One then appreciates why, when

*Source: American Academy of Pain Medicine, AAPM, http://www.painmed.org/PatientCenter/Facts_on_Pain.aspx

a healthcare professional is confronted with an apparently genuine pain complaint after having ruled out all possible physical causes of such pain, he/she is justified in referring the patient's complaint to an aberrant psychological state of mind. However, on the face of it, if psychological states of the mind are predominantly a function of brain activity (i.e. 'caused' by synaptic activity and neuronal firing), this brings the discussion back to the domain of the physical with the brain as a target organ of pathology.

The nuance here is extremely delicate; the editor of this book is especially cognizant of the current debate in the neurophilosophy field between Cartesian and Wittgenstanian camps, with ensuing debacles regarding mind-body dualism, the mereological fallcy, the concept of qualia, private experience, private language and language games, etc. [2,11,24] Far from being resolved, these emerging themes at the crossroads of philosophy and cognitive neuroscience are very relevant to pain researchers and ought to be considered in even the most basic empirical research at the levels of experimental planning and data interpretation. At the heart of the issue is *causation*. It is one thing to state that neuronal firing in the brain is a perquisite for unique mental states (i.e. without which cognition or consciousness is impossible), or that particular patterns of neuronal firing are highly correlated with unique mental states; it may also be tolerated to say that a particular pattern of firing among functionally connected brain networks *causes* a specific mental state. However, it is quite a leap of faith to suggest that the machinery for cognition or conscious perception can the shown in the brain (or parts of it). In other words, for example, to point at the somatosensory cortex and say "this is *where* sensation occurs" or "the somatosensory cortex engenders conscious perception of the sensory experience", such jargon amounts to nonsensical utterances. Attributing emotions such as fear, or sensory experiences such as pain, to specific brain "centers" is akin to Cartesian dualism. Statements such as "how does your brain perceive heat?" or "the brain that does not feel pain" have become common parlance in media and even top-ranked scientific journals. The brain does not "feel" or "perceive" anything, rather the human being does. This debacle has prompted at least one philosopher to accuse neuroscientists of making flagrantly "nonsensical claims".[24] This argument is succinctly encapsulated in the following quotation[2] (p. 142):

> The question of whether the brain is a possible subject of psychological attributes is distinct from the question whether the brain is the locus of those psychological attributes to which a corporeal location can intelligibly be assigned. Sensations such as pains and itches can be assigned a **location**[added emphasis]. The location of a pain is where the sufferer points, in the limb that he assuages, in the part of his body he describes as hurting- for it is these forms of pain **behavior**[added emphasis] that provide criteria for the location of pain. By contrast, thinking, believing, deciding, and wanting, for example, cannot be assigned a somatic location.

On **behavior**, simple and straightforward as this may be, a behavior that is indicative of pain cannot be taken as the ultimate criterion for pain in others (originally a Wittgensteinian claim central to the argument brought forth by Bennett and Hacker: "But doesn't what you say come to this: that there is no pain, for example, without pain-behaviour? It comes to this: only of a living human being and what resembles (behaves like) a living human being can one say: it has sensations; it sees; is blind; hears; is deaf; is conscious or unconscious." ([12] aphorism 281). I turn here to key counter-examples eloquently described by Nikola Grahek: the two most radical dissociation syndromes to be found in human experience, the first being complete dissociation of the sensory dimension of pain from its affective, cognitive, and behavioral components (or *pain without painfulness*, asymbolia), the second is absolute dissociation of the pain experience's affective components from its sensory-discriminative components (*painfulness without pain*).[4] Though most (if not all) pain researchers agree that pain is a complex experience comprising sensory-discriminative, emotional-cognitive, and behavioral components, which are normally tightly coupled, pain may become disconnected and, hence, *can* exist independently (i.e. with or without pain-indicative behavior).

On **location**, the issue is far from settled in the case of phantom pain, whereby clearly the patient's chief complaint is of an unpleasant sensation that is indeed referred to a body part, but that the part in question is amputated (i.e. non-existent in physical space). It becomes easy here (though not necessarily correct) to invoke brain mechanisms to explain the ontology of phantom pain, for where else could the pain "emanate" from? Here John Searle attempts to take a stab at it, taking the stance sensations, including pain, are all *in* the brain. Searle conjures a hypothesis, that is in part based on empirical evidence showing neuroplasticity in the cortex in the form of expanded receptive fields, concluding that the brain creates a body image, and the pain that we describe as being in the foot (though amputated), is in the body image that is in one's brain (or in the distorted body image in the exceptional case of phantom pain).[2]

Now Bennett and Hacker further assert "Which part of [someone's] brain is involved in [thinking, believing, etc.] is a further, important question about which neuroscientists are gradually learning more. But they are not learning where thinking, recollecting, or deciding occur—they are discovering which parts of the cortex are **causally** [added emphasis] implicated in a human being's thinking, recollecting, deciding"[2] (p142).

However, regarding **causality**, Bennett and Hacker back-peddle by claiming "if one opens the stomach, one can see the digestion of food going on there. But if one wants to see thinking going on, one should look at the Le Penseur, not at his brain. All his brain can show is what goes on there *while he is thinking*; all fMRI scanners can show is which parts of his brain are metabolizing more oxygen than others when [he] is thinking"[2] (p143). Note how Bennett and Hacker revert to the position of assigning a correlative function at best between brain mechanisms and cognition, not a causative one. Otherwise, they would have been comfortable in looking at the fMRI of someone who's thinking, identify the brain regions with increased BOLD signal, and say "this is the brain circuitry that is correlated with, *and* causing, thinking in that person" or, in other words, "this is the machinery that's required for thinking; it must operate thus to enable [him] to think." But they are apparently reluctant to accept that.

As Daniel Robinson exclaimed, "to get right to the main point, let us grant that if, indeed, all that marks out the domain of the mental is causally brought about by some set of 'states' in the brain, then, as the maxim goes, physics is complete and we can begin retooling philosophers for a second career"[2] (p. 177). He goes on to surmise that "I have little doubt but that the healthy and functional organization of the body, especially including the nervous system, constitutes the necessary *conditions* for what we are pleased to call our mental life […]. Nonetheless, the suggestion that excitable tissue causes all this would be nothing short of breathtaking in an age that had not already converted science into a species of rhetoric."

Perhaps not, I do agree, that science has not dwarfed into rhetoric. On the other hand, emerging evidence for the existence of measurable brain activity (whether by imaging or electrophysiological techniques) that is correlated with specific mental states, whose existence is sufficient to invoke that mental state, and which is reversed back to baseline with the disappearance of the mental state, to me is highly conducive for drawing the conclusion that, indeed, excitable tissue in the brain can, at least in principle, be causative of *certain* mental states. At this stage of pain research, however, I agree with the late Nikola Grahek, "we still do not have a fully satisfactory conceptual and neural model of pain that would explain all puzzling phenomena to be found in human pain experience and put pain under firm control"[4] (p. 5). However, he goes on to say, "we do know much more about pain than we knew only a few decades ago."

Our aim in this book is to contribute at least modestly to that knowledge, by showing empirical data resulting from scientific experimentation at the basic science and clinical levels. Between the flat-out rejection of assigning any anatomical locus for pain other than the body part that hurts, and the claim that all pains are in the brain (where in the brain remains unclear and how does the brain *sees that image within itself* remains a mystery), the reader is invited to seriously consider the merit of each standpoint and to reflect upon this on-going language game between Cartesians and Wittgensteinians, while the authors of this book were inclined to distance themselves from the debate (at least for now), in favor of *facts first*. As Daniel Dennett put it, anyone who has thought hard about pain knows that it can seem impossibly paradoxical and cryptic [4] (p. xiii).

References

1. Aydede M. In: Aydede M, ed. *Pain: New Essays on its Nature and the Methodology of its Study*. Cambridge: The MIT Press; 2005.
2. Bennett M, et al. *Neuroscience & Philosophy: Brain, Mind, & Language*. New York: Columbia University Press; 2007.
3. Fields HL. *Pain*. New York: McGraw-Hill; 1987.
4. Grahek N. *Feeling in Pain and Being in Pain*, 2nd ed. Cambridge: The MIT Press; 2001.
5. Morris DB. *The Culture of Pain*. Berkley: University of California Press; 1991.
6. Skevington SM. *Psychology of Pain*. New York: John Wiley & Sons; 1995.
7. Stiller R. *Pain: Why it Hurts, Where it Hurts, When it Hurts*. Nashville: Thomas Nelson Publishers; 1975.
8. IASP. In: Bogduk. HMN, ed. *Classification of Chronic Pain: Descriptions of Chronic Pain Syndromes and Definitions of Pain Terms* (2nd ed.). Seattle: IASP Press; 1994.
9. Axelrod FB, Gold-von Simson G. Hereditary sensory and autonomic neuropathies: types II, III, and IV. *Orphanet J Rare Dis*. 2007;2:39.
10. Wittgenstein L. *Tractatus Logico-Philosophicus*. New York: Routledge & Kegan Paul; 1961.
11. Kripke SA. *Wittgenstein: On Rules and Private Language*. Cambridge: Harvard University Press; 1982.
12. Anscombe GEM, Rhees R. *Philosophical Investigations*, 2nd ed. Oxford: Blackwell; 1953.
13. King T, et al. Unmasking the tonic-aversive state in neuropathic pain. *Nat Neurosci*. 2009;12(11):1364–1366.
14. Langford DJ, et al. Coding of facial expressions of pain in the laboratory mouse. *Nat Methods*. 2010;7(6):447–449.
15. Brand PW. Tenderizing the foot. *Foot Ankle Int*. 2003;24(6):457–461.
16. Brand PaYP. *Pain: The Gift Nobody Wants*. New York: Harper Collins; 1993.
17. Roy R. *The Social Context of the Chronic Pain Sufferer*. Toronto: The University of Toronto Press; 1992.
18. Liebeskind JC. Pain can kill. *Pain*. 1991;44(1):3–4.
19. Wall PD. In: Wall PD, Melzack. R, eds. *Textbook of pain* (4th ed.). New York: Churchill Livingstone; 1999.
20. Dworkin RH, et al. Evidence-based clinical trial design for chronic pain pharmacotherapy: a blueprint for ACTION. *Pain*. 2011;152(3 Suppl):S107–S115.
21. Latham J, Davis BD. The socioeconomic impact of chronic pain. *Disabil Rehabil*. 1994;16(1):39–44.
22. Sternbach RA. Pain and 'hassles' in the United States: findings of the Nuprin pain report. *Pain*. 1986;27(1):69–80.
23. Landmark T, et al. Estimating the prevalence of chronic pain: validation of recall against longitudinal reporting (the HUNT pain study). *Pain*. 2012;153(7):1368–1373.
24. Bennett MR, Hacker PMS. *Philosophical Foundations of Neuroscience*. Oxford: Blackwell Publishing; 2003.

2

Morphological Brain Changes in Chronic Pain: Mystery and Meaning

Eric Newman, Eric Moulton, Lino Becerra and David Borsook

P.A.I.N. Group, Boston Children's Hospital, Harvard Medical School, Waltham, Massachusetts, USA

INTRODUCTION

Chronic pain is defined as pain that lasts beyond the length of time necessary for the bodily insult or injury to heal. While there is no definitive length of time or level of pain that can be relied upon for diagnosis, most chronic pain syndromes are generally considered to last at least three months. A 2008 survey found that approximately 100 million American adults suffered from chronic pain.[1] The term chronic pain encompasses a variety of syndromes that include headache disorders, neuropathic pain conditions, irritable bowel syndrome (IBS), pain disorder, chronic prostatitis, chronic pelvic pain, and provoked vestibulodynia. In the past decade, it has become evident that chronic pain produces changes in the brain. Such changes suggest meaningful physiological processes that may provide insights into the unfolding of a chronic pain syndrome as well as how the brain may be remodeled in recovery.

METHODOLOGICAL APPROACHES TO MEASURES OF MORPHOMETRIC CHANGES IN THE CNS

Voxel-Based Morphometry

Unlike other morphometric measurements used in brain imaging studies that focus on volumes of unambiguous brain regions such as the hippocampi or ventricles, VBM is not biased to one particular region. It provides a method by which to study group differences in anatomy throughout the brain. At its core, VBM is a voxel-by-voxel comparison of grey matter (GM) concentration between subject groups. This measure is often described as GM density, but it is not equivalent to cytoarchitectonic density, so "concentration" is a better description. VBM consists of four distinct steps.[2] First, all the subjects' data must be transformed to the same stereotactic space to yield spatially normalized images. These images are then broken down into their constituent parts: GM, white matter (WM), cerebrospinal fluid (CSF), and background noise (3 classes).[3] The GM regions then need to be smoothed by convolving them with an isotropic Gaussian kernel. Essentially, spatial smoothing results in each voxel of the smoothed image containing the average concentration of GM from around the voxel. This renders the data more normally distributed as well as compensating for the inexact nature of the spatial normalization. Finally, statistical analysis is performed to localize regions of group differences. This yields a statistical parametric map that shows regions of significantly different GM concentration.

Diffusion MRI

Diffusion MRI (dMRI) is a MRI method that measures molecular diffusion in biological tissues. As molecules interact with many different obstacles as they diffuse throughout tissues, dMRI provides insight into the microscopic details of tissue architecture. There are various subtypes of dMRI, but for tissues with fibrous internal structures, such as white matter axons in brain tissue, diffusion tensor imaging (DTI) is used. Tissues with this type of fibrous internal structure exhibit anisotropy, or directionality of diffusion, meaning that water diffuses faster in the direction aligned with the internal structure than the direction perpendicular to it. This information can then be used to determine other characteristics of the tissue, including fractional anisotropy and connectivity.

Fractional Anisotropy

FA is a scalar value that describes the directionality of diffusion. It ranges from zero to one, with zero meaning that diffusion is isotropic (identical in all directions) and one meaning that diffusion is fully restricted in all directions except one. FA is a useful tool in determining WM structure, as its constituent parts exhibit specific directionality. For this reason, FA is thought to reflect fiber density, axonal diameter, and integrity of myelination.

Tractography

Each measure of FA corresponds to a specific direction of diffusion. This directional information can be extracted and presented visually, showing connections between different WM regions. This procedure is called tractography and it provides an invaluable *in vivo*, non-invasive approach to determine connectivity throughout the brain. One of the most important initial uses of tractography has been the localization of WM lesions[4,5] and tumors,[6,7] but it is becoming increasingly important in the understanding of WM changes associated with various disease states, including chronic pain.

THE BRAIN AND PLASTICITY

Adaptive Plasticity—Functional Drives Produce Structural Changes

What accounts for these structural differences? One of the major breakthroughs in the field of neuroscience was the discovery that the brain is adaptive or plastic and can change under physiological/healthy conditions. Early research in this field focused on functional effects of neuroplasticity through examination of cortical maps, cortical representations of the body based on somatotopic organization of sensory inputs to the cortex.[8,9] These studies reported that in the event of a serious bodily injury, such as an amputation or deafferentation, cortical maps for the areas affected by the injury were altered, in the sense that the representative body map remained intact, but the sensory inputs for the injured area would consequently come from other, usually adjacent inputs. In the somatosensory cortex for example, based on the classic Penfield homunculus,[10] as a result of the amputation of a hand, the cortical map could be altered so that input from the face would activate the "hand receptors" due to their juxtaposition on the representative body map. Neuroplasticity research significantly progressed with the advent of neuroimaging techniques that have provided evidence for altered structure and function of both cortical and subcortical regions. Since then, many studies have shown the correlation between training and brain structural changes. The two main quantitative measurements used in these studies have been gray matter (GM) differences (density, volume, thickness) via voxel-based morphometry (VBM) and white matter (WM) differences via fractional anisotropy (FA), which is thought to reflect WM characteristics such as fiber density, axonal diameter, and integrity of myelination.

Plasticity and Specialized Functional Activity

One of the first studies to examine structural plasticity in response to environmental demands was conducted by Maguire et al., in which MRI and VBM were used to compare the brain morphometry of experienced, professional taxi drivers to that of control subjects.[11,12] Increased posterior hippocampal volume was detected in the taxi drivers, and conversely, increased anterior hippocampal volume was detected in control subjects. Furthermore, the increased hippocampal volume in the taxi drivers was correlated with the amount of time spent in the profession. Similar results have been reported in studies of musicians' brain morphometry.[13–16] Compared to controls, musicians consistently exhibit increased GM volume and cortical thickness in brain areas associated with auditory processing, as well as increased FA in the posterior limb of the internal capsule, which contains fibers of the pyramidal tract as well as sensory fibers.

Plasticity—Cause or Consequence of Brain Activity

Although initial plasticity studies failed to determine whether the morphometric changes were the cause or the consequence of the training experience, subsequent longitudinal studies attempted to do so by examining brain morphometry of subjects prior to, during, and after the acquisition of a new skill, specifically juggling.[17,18] VBM and FA revealed no significant baseline structural differences between the two groups (jugglers and controls), yet in as few as seven days of training, the subjects in the juggler group showed GM thickening in the mid-temporal area and the left posterior intra-parietal sulcus (areas involved in processing of complex visual motion) as well as increased FA in WM underlying the right posterior intra-parietal sulcus. Rescanning the subjects after a period without training revealed that the GM expansion present in the second scan had diminished back to near-baseline levels, but the increased WM FA persisted. Together, these studies provided evidence for training-dependent GM and WM structural changes in healthy human brains.

Biological Changes in Gray Matter during Aging

Conversely, a large body of research has been conducted examining maladaptive neuroplasticity. The correlation between ageing and changes in brain morphometry has been noted for a long time. Research has shown that normal ageing amongst an adult population results in an average of 5.4 cm^3, or 0.5%, of whole-brain GM atrophy per year.[19] A defining study by Sowell and colleagues[20] used MRI with VBM and FA to examine cortical structure differences between age groups with subjects ranging from 7–87 years. Results showed decreased GM density in the most dorsal aspects of the frontal and parietal regions on both the lateral and interhemispheric surfaces, as well as in the orbitofrontal cortex, from age 7 to age 60, with little decline after age 60. GM density decreased approximately 32% in the superior frontal sulcus from age 7 to age 60, with only a 5% decrease between ages 40 and 87. GM density decreased 12% in the superior temporal sulcus from age 7 to age 60, with a 24% decrease between ages 40 and 87. The bilateral posterior temporal lobes and bilateral inferior parietal lobes exhibited a different pattern; a subtle increase in GM density until age 30 followed by a gradual decrease thereafter. Based on these findings, it was determined that in the most dorsal aspects of the parietal lobes, GM density reached its lowest point at 40–50 years, whereas in the frontal lobes, GM density reached its lowest point at 50–60 years. These results suggest that the association cortices of the frontal and parietal lobes show the most significant GM density loss early in life, while the primary auditory, visual, and anterior cingulate cortices show shallower GM decreases over the lifespan. Results also reported a steady increase of cerebrospinal fluid (CSF) volume with age, as well as that WM volume increased until age 43, after which time it began to decrease, showing that on average, WM volume was similar between the oldest and youngest subjects.

ALTERATIONS IN GRAY AND WHITE MATTER— PATHOPHYSIOLOGICAL PROCESSES

Taken together, the functional structural relationships—from development to old age, are a dynamic process. Both passive and active processes are capable of changing brain function and structure in health and disease. What are the physiological processes that account for these structural changes?

Possible Pathophysiological Mechanisms of Gray Matter Alterations

Neurogenesis: Neurogenesis presents an interesting possibility for a mechanism of brain structural changes. Preclinical research has shown that it is possible to genetically increase adult hippocampal neurogenesis.[21-23] Research suggests that 60–80% of young adult-born neurons undergo programmed cell death, which is at least partially caused by the pro-apoptotic gene *Bax*.[24] One study,[24] using a transgenic mouse line in which the *Bax* gene was repressed, reported increased amounts of adult-born neurons, as well as increased efficiency in differentiating between overlapping contextual representations, indicative of enhanced pattern separation. If this type of genetic approach can be used to increase adult neurogenesis in the hippocampus, perhaps it can be extended for use in the neocortex, although reports of adult neurogenesis in the neocortex are inconclusive.

Neuronal Morphology/Cerebral Vasculature Changes: Various training regimens have been shown to induce both neuronal morphological[25,26] and cerebral vasculature changes.[27] In a study[25] utilizing spatial learning via a water maze as a training paradigm, rats that were trained on the maze exhibited increased dendritic spine density on hippocampal CA1 pyramidal neurons, which the researchers determined to reflect an increased number of excitatory synapses per neuron associated with spatial learning. While preclinical results in the neocortex are varied and inconclusive, and clinical results are few and far between, these results nevertheless present a potential method for inducing GM changes. A large body of research examining dendritic spine density in the context of various disease states including Alzheimer's disease,[28–32] dementia,[28,32] Down's syndrome,[29,33–35] and schizophrenia[30,36,37] has reliably shown that patients exhibit decreased dendritic spine density as well as decreased total number of spines across a range of brain regions compared to controls. Regarding cerebral vasculature changes, preclinical studies have reliably shown increased vasculature branching and blood volume in animals on a physical exercise regimen,[23,38,39] and some research has reported increased blood flow via neuroimaging techniques in the hippocampus of humans on an exercise regimen.[23] Although most of the research in the field of cortical vasculature changes has been conducted in the context of differences in physical activity, the findings could potentially extend to other types of learning experiences, making vascular changes a potential mechanism for cortical thickness differences. While it is not agreed upon what these cerebral vasculature changes reflect, the training-induced vascular differences present another potential option for manipulating gray and white matter.

Non-Neuronal Cell Genesis and Morphology: Non-neuronal cells could also be responsible for GM morphometric changes. While mature neurons cannot divide, non-neuronal cells including astrocytes, oligodendrocyte progenitor cells (OPC's), glial cells, and endothelial cells, retain their ability to proliferate, presenting a possible mechanism of cortical thickening. Furthermore, experience-dependent gliogenesis and structural plasticity of other non-neuronal cells have been reported.[40] Astrocytes have also been shown to elicit various effects in response to neuronal

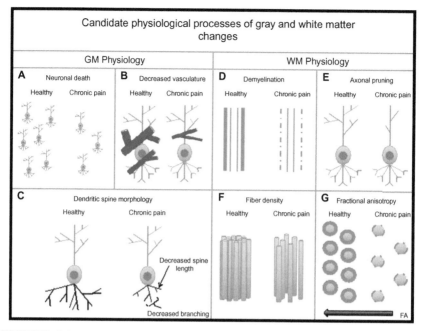

FIGURE 2.1 **Potential basis morphological changes.** A number of physiological mechanisms have been proposed to explain the gray and white matter changes visible in neuroimaging studies.[21–48] Decreased GM volume could be explained by **A** a decrease in the number of neurons due to neuronal death, **B** decreased vasculature, **C** and/or changes in dendritic spine morphology such as decreased spine length and decreased branching. Alterations in WM integrity could be explained by **D** demyelination of axons, **E** axonal pruning, and/or **F** decreased fiber density. These WM physiology alterations are thought to be measured by FA **G**. FA decreases as number of axons decreases, axons become less tightly packed, axonal diameter decreases, and myelination decreases.

activity,[41] as well as being implicated in chronic pain sensitization via potentiating synapse in the dorsal horn of the spinal cord,[42] suggesting another possible mechanism underlying changes in cortical thickness.

Possible Physiological Mechanisms of White Matter Alterations

Diffusion imaging measures are sensitive to various WM tissue properties, including myelination, axon diameter, packing density, axon permeability, and fiber geometry. Thus, these various tissue properties present possible mechanisms for the WM morphometry changes associated with chronic pain.

Myelination: Myelin has long been the focus for research into the physiology of various diseases, including Alzheimer's disease, Parkinson's disease, and other neurodegenerative conditions. Pre-clinical and post-mortem studies have shown myelination to be dynamic across the lifespan,[20,43] differing across brain regions, with increases in cerebral white matter characteristic of adulthood. Preclinical studies have also shown increased myelination in response to motor activity,[44] which presents myelination as an attractive physiological mechanism for WM changes, especially given the findings of WM structural changes in response to training. Ultimately, longitudinal histological and neuroimaging studies are required to provide more convincing evidence for myelination as an underlying physiological mechanism for WM changes observable using neuroimaging techniques.

Axonal Changes: Training has been shown to increase sprouting of mossy fiber axons in the hippocampus.[26] In preclinical studies of both spatial learning via a water maze[26] and forced and voluntary physical exercise,[45] results have shown that rats in the training groups exhibit increased hippocampal mossy fiber axon sprouting compared to rats in the control groups. Preclinical studies have also shown that activity-dependent competition with active axons plays a major role in axonal pruning. Using genetically altered mice in which certain populations of neurons in the hippocampal circuit are inactivated, results show that inactive axons are eliminated through competition with active axons.[46] Preclinical studies utilizing cortical damage models have also demonstrated altered cortico-cortical connectivity in response to training.[47,48] The results of these preclinical studies present axonal sprouting, pruning, and re-routing as strong potential options for inducing WM changes.

BRAIN CHANGES AND CHRONIC PAIN

Recent neuroimaging research, both preclinical and clinical, also suggests that the extended experience of chronic pain can negatively impact brain morphometry, specifically gray and white matter structure. An important preclinical study by Metz et al. used patch-clamp recordings and anatomical analysis of layer 2/3 pyramidal neurons in the contralateral medial prefrontal cortex of rats with the spared nerve injury (SNI) model of neuropathic pain and sham-operated rats.[49] As expected, the SNI rats exhibited lower tactile thresholds than the sham-operated rats, as demonstrated by the von Frey fiber test. The anatomical analysis showed significant morphological differences between the groups. Specifically, the basal dendrites of SNI rat neurons were longer and more branched than in the sham-operated rats and SNI rats exhibited selectively increased spine density in basal dendrites. The patch-clamp recordings showed significant functional differences between the groups. The NMDA/AMPA ratio showed a significantly larger fraction of current mediated by NMDA channels in the SNI rats, which was correlated with the rats' tactile threshold. This correlation existed in the operated paw, but not the contralateral paw, suggesting a relationship between the SNI pain-related NMDA/AMPA ratio and tactile threshold associated with allodynia of the operated paw. The medial prefrontal cortex in the rat model has been shown to be analogous to the prefrontal cortex in humans, which is involved in acute pain, pain unpleasantness, and anticipation of pain. Therefore, the morphological and functional changes found in the rat model suggest similar changes in chronic neuropathic pain in humans.

Alterations in Gray Matter Volume in CP

Ten distinct chronic pain syndromes have been reported to have brain morphometry changes: migraine, chronic tension-type headache, chronic back pain, phantom pain, fibromyalgia, irritable bowel syndrome, complex regional pain syndrome, pain disorder, chronic prostatitis/chronic pelvic pain, and provoked vestibulodynia. These are summarized in Table 2.1 and discussed in detail below.

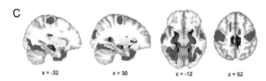

FIGURE 2.2   **Gray Matter Changes in Chronic Pain.** Cortical GM Differences Between Three Chronic Pain Conditions (CBP, CRPS, OA). **C** shows a comparison of areas of decreased GM density between CBP patients (red), CRPS patients (yellow), and OA patients (blue).[50]

TABLE 2.1   Regions of Decreased Gray Matter in Chronic Pain Syndromes

Syndrome	Cing. Cortex	Thalamus	Ins. Cortex	Temporal Lobes	Brain Stem	Ref.
Migraine	✓		✓	✓	✓	51–53
CTTH	✓		✓	✓	✓	54
CBP		✓		✓		55
Phantom Pain	✓				✓	56
FM		✓	✓			57,58
IBS	✓	✓	✓			59,60
CRPS			✓			61
Pain Disorder	✓		✓	✓	✓	62
CPP	✓	✓	✓			63

Migraine and Chronic Tension-Type Headache: According to the International Headache Society Classification ICHD-II,[64] other symptoms notwithstanding, a chronic migraineur presents with a headache not attributable to any other disorder occurring at least 15 days per month for at least three months. Although initial studies[65] reported no significant gray or white matter differences characteristic of chronic migraineurs, three later studies[51–53] reported reduced gray matter density in the anterior cingulate cortex, involved in pain-processing, anterior insulae, and temporal lobes, as well as increased gray matter density in the periaqueductal gray, involved in descending modulation of pain, and dorsolateral pons, compared to control subjects. It is important to note that the Rocca et al. study[51] had a small sample size and subjects presented with T2-visible lesions, something atypical of most migraineurs. In another study,[66] migraineurs exhibited thicker somatosensory cortex, which is crucially involved in noxious and nonnoxious somatosensory processing, compared to healthy controls. In a related chronic pain syndrome, chronic tension-type headache, significant gray matter morphometry differences were found.[54] Subjects with chronic tension-type headache showed decreased gray matter in the perigenual anterior, mid anterior, and right posterior cingulate cortex, bilateral anterior and posterior insula cortex, dorsal, rostral, and ventral pons, right posterior temporal lobe, orbitofrontal cortex, bilateral parahippocampus, and right cerebellum, most of which are involved in pain processing. Results also showed a continual positive correlation between years of headache duration and decreased gray matter in those areas.

Chronic Back Pain (CBP): According to the IASP guidelines,[67] chronic nonspecific back pain is defined as pain in the low back lasting longer than 12 weeks. CBP is one of the most common chronic pain syndromes and "In industrialized countries, low back pain (LBP) is the most common cause of activity limitation in persons younger than 45 years."[67] The first study to show brain morphometric changes in chronic pain was conducted by Apkarian et al., in which MRI and VBM were used to compare the brain structures of subjects suffering from CBP to control subjects, focusing on GM density and volume.[55] Results showed an approximately $30\,\text{cm}^3$ decrease in GM volume in the CBP group, corresponding to an 11% decrease, compared to controls. CBP patients showed significantly decreased GM density in both the right anterior thalamus and bilateral dorsolateral prefrontal cortex (DLPFC), both involved in pain-processing. The researchers concluded that the magnitude of the GM volume loss was equivalent to that of 10–20 years of normal ageing. Furthermore, they observed that the decreased GM volume was correlated with pain duration, which indicated a $1.3\,\text{cm}^3$ loss of GM for every year of chronic pain. Another VBM study expanded on these results.[68] In this study, CBP subjects showed a significant decrease in GM in the bilateral somatosensory cortex, right DLPFC, and right temporal lobe, as well as a GM increase in the bilateral putamen, involved in learning and various dopaminergic pathways, and left posterior thalamus, a major source of nociceptive inputs to the cortex. Although the thalamic GM changes reported in the two studies[55,68] oppose each other, together, the results of these two studies suggest that the pathophysiology of chronic pain involves thalamocortical processes.

Phantom Limb Pain: Phantom pain is a perfect example of maladaptive neuroplasticity. Decades of research in the field have shown that somatosensory maps can be significantly altered in response to an amputation or deafferentation, leading to chronic pain.[69–72] And, it has recently been demonstrated that changes in cortical structure underlie these functional, topographical changes. A study by Draganski et al. examined the brain morphometry of unilateral amputees versus control subjects using MRI and VBM.[56] The results showed that the amputees exhibited decreased GM in the posterolateral thalamus contralateral to the amputation site and that these GM differences were positively correlated with length of time since the amputation but not correlated with the presence of phantom pain, suggesting that these morphometric changes reflect a structural correlate of the lost sensory input from the amputated area. Decreases in GM in the cingulate cortex and brain stem however, were correlated with phantom pain.

Fibromyalgia (FM): FM is a chronic pain syndrome in which sufferers present with chronic body-wide pain as well as tenderness in muscles, joints, and other soft tissues. Two important studies have been conducted looking at brain morphometry changes resulting from chronic FM pain.[57,58] In both studies, MRI and VBM were used to compare GM between FM subjects and control subjects. One study[57] found that FM subjects showed decreased GM density in the left parahippocampal gyrus, involved in stress, bilateral mid/posterior cingulate gyrus, left insula, and medial frontal cortex, all of which are involved in pain processing. The other study[58] found that FM subjects showed decreased GM in the right superior temporal gyrus and left posterior thalamus, as well as an increase in GM in the left orbitofrontal cortex, involved in the affective aspects of pain, left cerebellum, and bilateral striatum, compared to the control subjects.

Irritable Bowel Syndrome (IBS): Other symptoms notwithstanding, typical IBS sufferers present with moderate to severe abdominal pain at least three days a month for at least three consecutive months, and like the other chronic pain syndromes, IBS has been shown to change the brain morphometry of its sufferers. Two main studies[59,60] have used MRI and VBM to observe differences in brain morphometry between IBS subjects and control subjects. The studies showed a positive correlation between IBS and decreased GM in the cingulate cortex, thalamus/basal ganglia, hypothalamus, which the researchers suggest may be related to the association between IBS, stress, and the hypothalamic-pituitary-adrenal axis, and insula cortex. Furthermore, one study[59] showed that cortical thinning in the insula was present in short-term IBS subjects, but insular thickness was near normal in long-term IBS subjects.

Complex Regional Pain Syndrome (CRPS): CRPS is a debilitating syndrome characterized by intense burning pain, which begins at a point of injury and spreads, becoming more severe over time. There are two types of CRPS: CRPS I, which is a chronic nerve disorder that occurs after an injury, and CRPS II, which is caused by an injury to the nerve.[73] One recent study has shown the correlation between CRPS and abnormal brain morphometry.[61] This study used MRI and VBM to examine the GM structural differences in the brains of CRPS subjects compared to control subjects. The results showed that CRPS subjects displayed GM atrophy in the right insula, related to pain duration and intensity, right ventromedial prefrontal cortex (VMPFC), related to emotional decision-making, and the nucleus accumbens. It is important to note that despite these specific findings, results also showed that unlike the studies looking at chronic back pain[55,68] and fibromyalgia,[57,58] whole brain GM was similar between CRPS subjects and control subjects.

Pain Disorder: As defined by the American Psychiatric Association's Diagnostic and Statistical Manual and Mental Disorders, fourth Edition (DSM-IV),[74] chronic pain disorder is characterized by pain in one or more anatomical sites lasting longer than six months that cannot be accounted for by any physiological process, injury, or physical disorder. The onset, severity, exacerbation, and maintenance of this pain have been shown to have a strong correlation with psychological factors. A study[62] examining GM changes of chronic pain disorder patients using MRI and VBM reported significantly decreased GM density in the prefrontal cortex, specifically the VMPFC, orbitofrontal cortex, and middle frontal and superior medial frontal cortex, anterior and posterior cingulate cortex, parahippocampal cortex, inferior temporal cortex, and cerebellum.

Chronic Prostatitis/Chronic Pelvic Pain (CPP): CPP in women is characterized by non-cyclic pain lasting longer than six months located in the pelvis, abdomen, lumbosacral back, and/or buttocks.[75] CPP is either present on its own or in association with endometriosis. One study examined GM volume differences in patients with CPP and endometriosis-associated CPP.[63] Patients with endometriosis-associated CPP showed decreased GM volume in the left thalamus, left middle frontal gyrus, bilateral mid cingulate cortex, right putamen and right insular cortex, as well as increased GM volume in the left amygdala compared to healthy controls. CPP patients showed decreased GM volume only in the left thalamus.

Chronic prostatitis/chronic pelvic pain in men is a chronic pain condition characterized by pelvic or perineal pain lasting longer than three months with urinary tract infection ruled out as a cause.[75] A study in male chronic prostatitis/CPP patients utilized fMRI, VBM, and WM connectivity measures to examine brain functional and anatomical changes.[76] Functionally, patients showed functional activation in the right anterior insula, which was correlated with clinical pain intensity. Anatomically, no GM volume differences were reported, but GM density in the anterior insula and anterior cingulate cortices were positively correlated with pain intensity and extent of pain chronicity. In addition, patients exhibited an abnormal correlation between WM anisotropy and neocortical GM volume.

Provoked Vestibulodynia (PVD): PVD is a common form of chronic vulvar pain. The underlying pathophysiological mechanisms are unknown. In a study[77] examining GM density changes in PVD patients using MRI and VBM, no whole-brain GM volume differences were reported, but significantly increased GM density in patients was reported in the basal ganglia, substantia nigra, globus pallidus, hippocampus proper, right parahippocampal gyrus, and left caudate nucleus. These brain regions are known to be involved in pain modulation as well as the emotional and affective aspects of pain. These reported GM density increases are in stark contrast with the pattern of decreased GM density and volume that is present in the other chronic pain conditions.[51-76] The researchers hypothesize that this significant difference is likely related to the difference in the nature of the conditions, as PVD is a provoked condition while the other conditions are relatively spontaneous.

Gray Matter Changes—A Common Signature of Chronic Pain

The results of the brain morphometry studies for all these chronic pain syndromes provide insights to understanding that plasticity of brain structure plays a key role in the chronicity of pain. It is unclear whether this is adaptive or maladaptive. Furthermore, it can be seen that many of the areas that experience structural changes concomitant with chronic nociceptive input, such as the DLPFC, cingulate cortex, thalamus, orbitofrontal cortex, and insula cortex, do so across a variety of chronic pain syndromes, which suggests that there may be a common "brain signature" of chronic pain patients.

Correlation of Functional Changes and Gray Matter Changes

Functional changes have also been demonstrated in chronic pain patients. Research into the default mode network (DMN), an activation network involved in the functions of a resting brain state, has shed some initial light on functional differences associated with chronic pain.[78] The DMN represents co-activation of low frequency activations in a distributed network of cortical regions that is observed in the resting state or task-negative network. DMN functional changes have been used to characterize various brain states, such as those of neurodegenerative diseases and medicinal effects. In a study of chronic lower back pain (CLBP) subjects pre/post treatment, the researchers examined the subjects' functional characteristics in addition to the morphometric changes.[79] To do this, subjects were administered the Multi-Source Interference Task (MSIT), in which subjects responded to a stimulus on a screen in the MRI using a three-button control box. The task had a motor control task, in which an asterisk moved across the screen in sequential order, an easy level, and a difficult level. For contrast, "In the most difficult level of the task, the target character is a number displayed with other numbers of varying size."

Functional MRI's (fMRI) were obtained as the subjects completed the MSIT. The first MSIT with fMRI was conducted at baseline, the second at six weeks post-treatment, for which only a small subset of subjects returned, and the third at six months post-treatment, for which most subjects returned. The MSIT results showed no between-group differences or pre/post-treatment differences in terms of performance. However, the fMRI results showed that the CLBP subjects exhibited a greater area of task-related activations and fewer task-related deactivations when

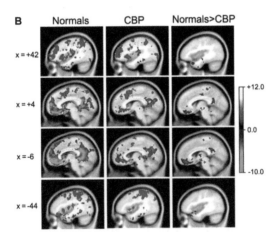

FIGURE 2.3   **Default mode networks (DMN) in chronic pain.** Activation differences between CBP patients and healthy controls. Compared to healthy controls, CBP patients exhibit deactivation in the medial prefrontal cortex, amygdala, and posterior cingulate/precuneus during an attention task.[78]

compared to control subjects. In the pre-treatment scan, CLBP subjects exhibited more task-related activation in a number of areas, including the left DLPFC. Post-treatment, CLBP subjects exhibited deactivation in the left DLPFC compared to pre-treatment, closer to control values. When looking at the data from baseline to six months post-treatment, an interesting pattern emerges. At six weeks post-treatment, the CLBP subjects exhibited a significant functional change towards control levels, while no significant morphometric GM changes were exhibited, and at six-months post treatment, the CLBP subjects exhibited both significant functional and morphometric GM changes. Although the data set for the six weeks post-treatment test was small, these results suggest that functional changes occur before anatomical changes occur and therefore offer a potential avenue for early treatment measures in the course of chronic pain syndrome.

Alterations in White Matter Tracts in CP

While a large body of research has focused on the GM changes associated with various disease states, comparatively fewer studies have examined WM changes in the context of disease pathology, and even fewer have examined them in the context of chronic pain syndromes. A number of studies have consistently demonstrated the presence of WM lesions associated with neurodegenerative diseases, including white matter disease,[80,81] Alzheimer's disease,[82–85] dementia,[86,87] and multiple sclerosis,[88,89] as well as psychological disorders including depression[85] and schizophrenia.[90] Three important studies have been conducted

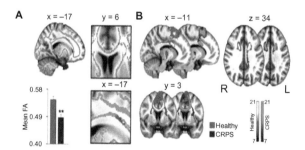

FIGURE 2.4   White matter changes in chronic pain. Comparison of white matter integrity (FA and tractography) between CRPS patients and healthy controls. **A** shows decreased FA in CRPS patients in a cluster within the left callosal fiber tract, adjacent to the anterior cingulate cortex. **B** shows probabilistic tractography using the region of decreased FA white matter as the seed. CRPS patients exhibited decreased probability of connections between the seed and the posterior cingulate as well as decreased connectivity between the seed and the left hemisphere.[61]

examining WM changes in the context of chronic pain, specifically in CRPS, migraine, and IBS.

The CRPS study[61] used FA and connectivity methods (Sholl analysis and probabilistic tractography) to examine WM differences. Regarding FA, the researchers demonstrated that whole brain skeletal FA did not differ between groups, but they did report a positive correlation between whole brain skeletal FA and GM volume in healthy subjects that was not present in CRPS subjects, suggesting a general structural relationship disruption between gray and white matter in CRPS. The researchers also reported that CRPS subjects exhibited lower FA values in a cluster within the left callosal fiber tract, adjacent to the anterior cingulate cortex, which is involved in pain processing. Regarding connectivity, CRPS subjects exhibited a prominent decrease in the probability of connections to the posterior cingulate area, as well as lower average number of connections at long distances in the left hemisphere and lower total number of connections in the left hemisphere. These results support the hypothesis that CRPS sufferers have altered WM structure and connectivity.

The migraine study[91] used the same methods to examine WM structure and connectivity differences between migraine subjects and control subjects. The researchers reported that the migraine subjects showed reduced FA in the right frontal WM cluster. Furthermore, probabilistic tractography showed connections between this area of WM atrophy and other parts of the pain network, including the orbitofrontal cortex, insula, thalamus, and dorsal midbrain. These results suggest maladaptive plastic changes and altered WM integrity (as measured by anisotropy) in migraine patients.

The IBS study[92] used DTI and FA as measures of WM integrity in IBS patients. Compared to controls, patients exhibited increased FA in the fornix and external capsule adjacent to the right posterior insula. The fornix is a region of white matter that connects the hippocampus to the hypothalamus and thus, integrates autonomic and emotional brain functions. As the hypothalamus receives nociceptive input via the spinohypothalamic pathway, the fornix may play a role in nociception due to its ability to sensitize the limbic system to nociceptive input. Therefore, the researchers suggest that the increased fornix FA in the IBS patients could be indicative of increased spinohypothalamic nociceptive fibers. As the hypothalamus is also involved in emotions and stress responses, the fornix could be involved in the emotional, affective aspects of pain. The insula is fundamentally entwined in the pain-processing system, with the right posterior insula being involved in visceral nociception. Thus, the increased FA of the external capsule adjacent to the right posterior insula reported in the IBS patients is consistent with previous findings suggesting abnormal insular activity in IBS.

BRAIN TARGETS FOR TREATMENT

Reversal of Gray Matter Changes

While brain morphometry changes associated with chronic pain are a serious concern, they are not permanent. Two recent studies used MRI and VBM to examine the effect of treatment on brain morphometry in subjects with chronic pain syndromes. One study[79] examined lower back pain (CLBP) pre and post-treatment, compared to control subjects. At baseline, the CLBP subjects exhibited decreased cortical thickness in the left DLPFC, bilateral anterior insular/frontal operculum, left mid/posterior insula, left primary somatosensory cortex (S1), left medial temporal lobe, and right anterior cingulate cortex compared to control subjects. CLBP subjects were then administered treatment, either in the form of spine surgery or zygapophysial (facet) joint blocks. Six months post-treatment, the CLBP subjects were scanned again. Remarkably, the second scan showed an increase in cortical thickness in all areas. However, all areas other than the DLPFC were still thinner than those of the control subjects.

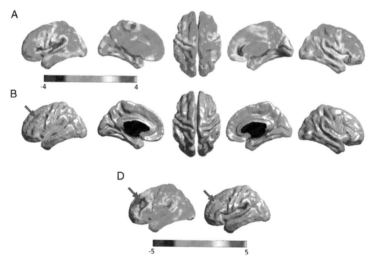

FIGURE 2.5 Comparison of cortical thickness between CLBP patients and healthy controls following treatment. **A** shows areas of thinner cortex in CLBP patients as shown by positive t-values (red/yellow). **B** shows random-field theory-based cluster-corrected maps of cortical thinning in CLBP patients compared to healthy controls. **D** shows uncorrected and corrected statistical maps for patients who responded to treatment. Arrows point to the cortical thickening that took place in the left DLPFC.[79]

Likewise, reports have examined brain GM differences between subjects with chronic pain due to primary hip osteoarthritis (OA) and control subjects.[93] The MRI and VBM showed decreased GM in the OA subjects in the anterior cingulate cortex, right insular cortex and operculum, DLPFC, amygdala, and brainstem. A small subset of the OA subjects was subsequently treated with total hip replacement surgery. Four months post-treatment, the OA subjects, all of which were completely pain free, returned for another MRI. The results showed a GM increase in the DLPFC, anterior cingulate cortex, amygdala, and brainstem.

While the results of these studies show that the brain atrophy associated with chronic pain can be at least somewhat reversed with treatment, they also prove to be important for another reason. Throughout the various studies examining brain morphometry changes associated with chronic pain, researchers have ultimately faced the question of whether these brain morphometry changes were a cause or a consequence of chronic pain. Seminowicz and colleagues found that the GM decreases of chronic pain subjects are at least partly reversible with treatment, suggesting that the structural changes must be the consequence of the chronic nociceptive transmission characteristic of these chronic pain syndromes. These gray and white matter characteristics provide potential options for measures of treatment efficacy. As these brain morphometry changes are dynamic and well defined over a relatively short period of time, studies of drugs targeted for chronic pain conditions should include VBM, FA, and other measures of WM tract integrity as measures of treatment's efficacy.

BIOMARKER IN CHRONIC PAIN: STRUCTURAL-FUNCTIONAL RELATIONSHIPS

The treatment of chronic pain conditions has always challenged clinicians. This is in large part due to the lack of biomarkers for chronic pain. But, with the recent studies of the functional and structural characteristics of chronic pain states, especially the finding that functional activation normalizes before structure does following treatment, new light is being shed on possible biomarkers. Looking at the functional or structural characteristics in isolation is insufficient as these changes are dynamic and highly intertwined. Studies examining concomitant functional and structural changes in the context of specific disease states are necessary to understand the complex relationship between the two and develop effective biomarkers.

Thus far, only a few studies have examined this relationship in the context of chronic pain conditions, specifically migraine,[94] cluster headache,[95] trigeminal neuropathic pain (TNP),[96] IBS,[60] and CBP.[97] The methods vary between studies but generally MRI with VBM is used to examine structural differences and either fMRI or PET and/or functional connectivity analysis is used to examine functional differences. Areas of concomitant structural and functional changes have been reported in all of these studies, notably the somatosensory cortex, cingulate cortex, insular cortex, DLPFC, hypothalamus, thalamus, nucleus accumbens, and basal ganglia. As all of these regions are involved in either the pain-processing or affective aspects of chronic pain conditions, the results agree with previous findings examining separate structural and functional changes associated with chronic pain. Furthermore, the study of CBP patients[97] revealed significant structural and functional differences between recovering sub-acute chronic back pain patients (SBPr) and persistent sub-acute chronic back pain patients (SBPp) which provides insight into the *chronification* of pain. Namely, SBPp patients exhibited significantly decreased GM density in pain-processing regions and significantly increased functional connectivity between regions involved in the pain-processing and affective aspects of chronic pain. The findings reported in these studies provide important insight into possible biomarkers of chronic pain, but more research utilizing neuroimaging techniques, both structural and functional, is necessary to determine the ultimate significance of these findings as well as to expand the results to other pain conditions.

Effects of Opioid Dependence on Brain Structure and Function

While a substantial body of research has reported structural and functional alterations in the brains of illicit opioid-dependent individuals, little research has been conducted on the structural and functional effects of prescription opioid-dependence on the brain. In a defining study by Upadhyay et al.,[98] structural differences between opioid-dependent individuals and healthy controls were examined using MRI with VBM and DTI with FA while functional differences were examined using functional connectivity. Structurally, prescription opioid-dependent subjects exhibited decreased GM volume in the bilateral amygdala as well as significantly decreased FA in amygdala axonal pathways and the internal and external capsules compared to healthy controls. Functionally, prescription opioid-dependent subjects exhibited significantly decreased functional connectivity in the insula, amygdala, and nucleus accumbens. More specifically, with the insula as the seed region, prescription opioid-dependent subjects exhibited decreased functional connectivity to the anterior cingulate and putamen. Furthermore, it was determined that the duration of prescription opioid-dependence was positively correlated with more drastic changes in functional connectivity. Given the functions of the various brain regions affected both structurally and functionally

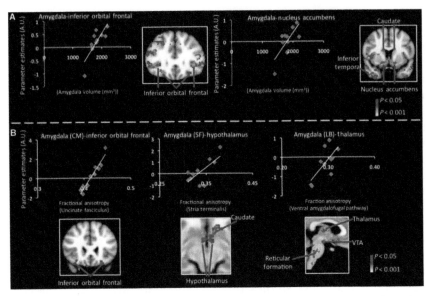

FIGURE 2.6   **Effects of Chronic Opioids on Brain Structure/Function.** Inter-dependent amygdalar structural and functional changes observed in prescription opioid-dependent subjects. **A** shows the inter-dependent relationship between amygdalar volume and functional connectivity. **B** shows the inter-dependent relationship between amygdalar WM FA and functional connectivity.[98]

by prescription opioid-dependence, the results suggest that prescription opioid-dependence negatively effects the regulation of affect, impulse control, reward, and motivation.

Sex-Dependent Structural and Functional Differences in Migraine

Researchers have long been aware of the difference in prevalence of migraine between the sexes. Females are twice as likely to suffer from migraine than males. However, the mechanisms responsible for this difference are not well understood. New evidence suggests that the female migraine brain is structurally and functionally different than the male migraine brain. This recent study[99] used MRI with automated parcellation tools to examine volumetric GM differences between the sexes and fMRI with noxious thermal stimulation as well as functional connectivity to examine functional differences between the sexes.

Structurally, female migraineurs exhibited greater cortical thickness in the left superiorfrontal, right caudal middle frontal gyrus, right supramarginal gyrus, bilateral precentral gyrus, left insula, and bilateral precuneus compared to male migraineurs. Functionally, in response to the noxious thermal stimulation female migraineurs exhibited stronger positive BOLD responses in the bilateral caudate, contralateral superior temporal, ipsilateral superior frontal, and contralateral precuneus, contralateral posterior cingulate, and brainstem regions. Conversely, male migraineurs exhibited stronger BOLD responses in the bilateral insula, contralateral primary somatosensory cortex, and contralateral putamen. Multiple areas, including the contralateral nucleus accumbens, contralateral amygdala, and bilateral hippocampus, showed deactivation in response to the noxious thermal stimulation and in both the amygdala and hippocampus, the negative response was stronger in female migraineurs. Regarding the functional connectivity analysis, brain regions that showed significant cortical thickness differences, including the insular cluster and precuneus cluster, were used as seed regions. Female migraineurs exhibited stronger negative functional connectivity between the insula and the primary somatosensory cortex, posterior cingulate, precuneus, and temporal pole and between the precuneus and the primary somatosensory cortex and amygdala.

To date, few studies have focused on sex-dependent differences in pain conditions despite the significant difference in prevalence between the sexes in many chronic pain conditions. This study provides significant evidence of inter-dependent sex-related structural and functional brain differences in a very prevalent, well-studied pain condition.

CONCLUSIONS

Recent preclinical and clinical research has shown that consistent nociceptive input, due to the chronicity of pain, can result in changes in brain morphometry, specifically changes in cortical and subcortical GM thickness, WM atrophy and connectivity, and dendritic spine morphology and function in a number of important areas, most of which are involved in either sensory or emotional and affective aspects of pain. These changes have been found across a number of chronic pain syndromes, suggesting a common "brain signature" of chronic pain. Furthermore, it has been demonstrated that with treatment for chronic pain, not only does brain activation return towards normal patterns, but resultant brain morphometry deficits at least partially reverse. Therefore, it has been determined that the brain morphometry changes associated with chronic pain are the consequence of the consistent nociceptive input, rather than the cause. These findings suggest that the treatment of chronic pain follows an observable and predictable progression, from removal of the painful stimulus/injury to normalization of altered brain function to reversal of gray and white matter atrophy and normalization of WM connectivity. The pathophysiological mechanisms underlying the morphometric changes are not well known, but a few possibilities have been proposed. These findings present gray and white matter characteristics as potential measures of treatment efficacy. More research in this field is necessary but even these preliminary findings provide hope that one day these debilitating conditions can be managed effectively using preventative, personalized treatment methods.

References

1. Tsang A, Von Korff M, Lee S, et al. Common chronic pain conditions in developed and developing countries: gender and age differences and comorbidity with depression-anxiety disorders. *J Pain*. 2008;9(10):883–891.
2. Ashburner J, Friston KJ. Voxel-based morphometry—the methods. *Neuroimage*. 2000;11(6 Pt 1):805–821.
3. Ashburner J, Friston K. Multimodal image coregistration and partitioning—a unified framework. *Neuroimage*. 1997;6(3):209–217.
4. Chen X, Weigel D, Ganslandt O, Buchfelder M, Nimsky C. Diffusion tensor imaging and white matter tractography in patients with brainstem lesions. *Acta Neurochir (Wien)*. 2007;149(11):1117–1131. [discussion 1131].
5. Clark CA, Barrick TR, Murphy MM, Bell BA. White matter fiber tracking in patients with space-occupying lesions of the brain: a new technique for neurosurgical planning? *Neuroimage*. 2003;20(3):1601–1608.
6. Akai H, Mori H, Aoki S, et al. Diffusion tensor tractography of gliomatosis cerebri: fiber tracking through the tumor. *J Comput Assist Tomogr*. 2005;29(1):127–129.
7. Schonberg T, Pianka P, Hendler T, Pasternak O, Assaf Y. Characterization of displaced white matter by brain tumors using combined DTI and fMRI. *Neuroimage*. 2006;30(4):1100–1111.
8. Hubel DH, Wiesel TN. Receptive fields, binocular interaction and functional architecture in the cat's visual cortex. *J Physiol*. 1962;160:106–154.
9. Merzenich MM, Nelson RJ, Kaas JH, et al. Variability in hand surface representations in areas 3b and 1 in adult owl and squirrel monkeys. *J Comp Neurol*. 1987;258(2):281–296.
10. Penfield W, Jasper HH. *Epilepsy and the Functional Anatomy of the Human Brain*, 1st ed. Boston: Little; 1954.
11. Maguire EA, Gadian DG, Johnsrude IS, et al. Navigation-related structural change in the hippocampi of taxi drivers. *Proc Natl Acad Sci U S A*. 2000;97(8):4398–4403.
12. Maguire EA, Spiers HJ, Good CD, Hartley T, Frackowiak RS, Burgess N. Navigation expertise and the human hippocampus: a structural brain imaging analysis. *Hippocampus*. 2003;13(2):250–259.
13. Bengtsson SL, Nagy Z, Skare S, Forsman L, Forssberg H, Ullen F. Extensive piano practicing has regionally specific effects on white matter development. *Nat Neurosci*. 2005;8(9):1148–1150.
14. Luders E, Gaser C, Jancke L, Schlaug G. A voxel-based approach to gray matter asymmetries. *Neuroimage*. 2004;22(2):656–664.
15. Han Y, Yang H, Lv YT, et al. Gray matter density and white matter integrity in pianists' brain: a combined structural and diffusion tensor MRI study. *Neurosci Lett*. 2009;459(1):3–6.
16. Scholz J, Klein MC, Behrens TE, Johansen-Berg H. Training induces changes in white-matter architecture. *Nat Neurosci*. 2009;12(11):1370–1371.
17. Draganski B, Gaser C, Busch V, Schuierer G, Bogdahn U, May A. Neuroplasticity: changes in grey matter induced by training. *Nature*. 2004;427(6972):311–312.

18. Driemeyer J, Boyke J, Gaser C, Buchel C, May A. Changes in gray matter induced by learning—revisited. *PLoS One*. 2008;3(7):e2669.

19. Resnick SM, Pham DL, Kraut MA, Zonderman AB, Davatzikos C. Longitudinal magnetic resonance imaging studies of older adults: a shrinking brain. *J Neurosci*. 2003;23(8):3295–3301.

20. Sowell ER, Peterson BS, Thompson PM, Welcome SE, Henkenius AL, Toga AW. Mapping cortical change across the human life span. *Nat Neurosci*. 2003;6(3):309–315.

21. Sahay A, Scobie KN, Hill AS, et al. Increasing adult hippocampal neurogenesis is sufficient to improve pattern separation. *Nature*. 2011;472(7344):466–470.

22. Cameron HA, McKay RD. Adult neurogenesis produces a large pool of new granule cells in the dentate gyrus. *J Comp Neurol*. 2001;435(4):406–417.

23. Pereira AC, Huddleston DE, Brickman AM, et al. An *in vivo* correlate of exercise-induced neurogenesis in the adult dentate gyrus. *Proc Natl Acad Sci USA*. 2007;104(13):5638–5643.

24. Sun W, Winseck A, Vinsant S, Park OH, Kim H, Oppenheim RW. Programmed cell death of adult-generated hippocampal neurons is mediated by the proapoptotic gene Bax. *J Neurosci*. 2004;24(49):11205–11213.

25. Moser MB, Trommald M, Andersen P. An increase in dendritic spine density on hippocampal CA1 pyramidal cells following spatial learning in adult rats suggests the formation of new synapses. *Proc Natl Acad Sci USA*. 1994;91(26):12673–12675.

26. Ramirez-Amaya V, Escobar ML, Chao V, Bermudez-Rattoni F. Synaptogenesis of mossy fibers induced by spatial water maze overtraining. *Hippocampus*. 1999;9(6):631–636.

27. Olson AK, Eadie BD, Ernst C, Christie BR. Environmental enrichment and voluntary exercise massively increase neurogenesis in the adult hippocampus via dissociable pathways. *Hippocampus*. 2006;16(3):250–260.

28. Catala I, Ferrer I, Galofre E, Fabregues I. Decreased numbers of dendritic spines on cortical pyramidal neurons in dementia. A quantitative Golgi study on biopsy samples. *Hum Neurobiol*. 1988;6(4):255–259.

29. Ferrer I, Gullotta F. Down's syndrome and Alzheimer's disease: dendritic spine counts in the hippocampus. *Acta Neuropathol*. 1990;79(6):680–685.

30. Garey LJ, Ong WY, Patel TS, et al. Reduced dendritic spine density on cerebral cortical pyramidal neurons in schizophrenia. *J Neurol Neurosurg Psychiatr*. 1998;65(4):446–453.

31. Knobloch M, Mansuy IM. Dendritic spine loss and synaptic alterations in Alzheimer's disease. *Mol Neurobiol*. 2008;37(1):73–82.

32. Mehraein P, Yamada M, Tarnowska-Dziduszko E. Quantitative study on dendrites and dendritic spines in Alzheimer's disease and senile dementia. *Adv Neurol*. 1975;12:453–458.

33. Becker LE, Armstrong DL, Chan F. Dendritic atrophy in children with Down's syndrome. *Ann Neurol*. 1986;20(4):520–526.

34. Suetsugu M, Mehraein P. Spine distribution along the apical dendrites of the pyramidal neurons in Down's syndrome. A quantitative Golgi study. *Acta Neuropathol*. 1980;50(3):207–210.

35. Kaufmann WE, Moser HW. Dendritic anomalies in disorders associated with mental retardation. *Cereb Cortex*. 2000;10(10):981–991.

36. Glantz LA, Lewis DA. Decreased dendritic spine density on prefrontal cortical pyramidal neurons in schizophrenia. *Arch Gen Psychiatr*. 2000;57(1):65–73.

37. Sweet RA, Henteleff RA, Zhang W, Sampson AR, Lewis DA. Reduced dendritic spine density in auditory cortex of subjects with schizophrenia. *Neuropsychopharmacology*. 2009;34(2):374–389.

38. Rhyu IJ, Bytheway JA, Kohler SJ, et al. Effects of aerobic exercise training on cognitive function and cortical vascularity in monkeys. *Neuroscience*. 2010;167(4):1239–1248.

39. Swain RA, Harris AB, Wiener EC, et al. Prolonged exercise induces angiogenesis and increases cerebral blood volume in primary motor cortex of the rat. *Neuroscience*. 2003;117(4):1037–1046.

40. Dong WK, Greenough WT. Plasticity of nonneuronal brain tissue: roles in developmental disorders. *Ment Retard Dev Disabil Res Rev.* 2004;10(2):85–90.

41. Wang X, Takano T, Nedergaard M. Astrocytic calcium signaling: mechanism and implications for functional brain imaging. *Methods Mol Biol.* 2009;489:93–109.

42. Ji RR, Kawasaki Y, Zhuang ZY, Wen YR, Decosterd I. Possible role of spinal astrocytes in maintaining chronic pain sensitization: review of current evidence with focus on bFGF/JNK pathway. *Neuron Glia Biol.* 2006;2(4):259–269.

43. Bartzokis G, Lu PH, Tingus K, et al. Lifespan trajectory of myelin integrity and maximum motor speed. *Neurobiol Aging.* 2010;31(9):1554–1562.

44. Ullen F. Is activity regulation of late myelination a plastic mechanism in the human nervous system?. *Neuron Glia Biol.* 2009;5(1-2):29–34.

45. Toscano-Silva M, Gomes da Silva S, Scorza FA, Bonvent JJ, Cavalheiro EA, Arida RM. Hippocampal mossy fiber sprouting induced by forced and voluntary physical exercise. *Physiol Behav.* 2010;101(2):302–308.

46. Yasuda M, Johnson-Venkatesh EM, Zhang H, Parent JM, Sutton MA, Umemori H. Multiple forms of activity-dependent competition refine hippocampal circuits *in vivo*. *Neuron.* 2011;70(6):1128–1142.

47. Johansen-Berg H. Structural plasticity: rewiring the brain. *Curr Biol.* 2007;17(4): R141–R144.

48. Dancause N, Barbay S, Frost SB, et al. Extensive cortical rewiring after brain injury. *J Neurosci.* 2005;25(44):10167–10179.

49. Metz AE, Yau HJ, Centeno MV, Apkarian AV, Martina M. Morphological and functional reorganization of rat medial prefrontal cortex in neuropathic pain. *Proc Natl Acad Sci USA.* 2009;106(7):2423–2428.

50. Baliki MN, Schnitzer TJ, Bauer WR, Apkarian AV. Brain morphological signatures for chronic pain. *PLoS One.* 2011;6(10):e26010.

51. Rocca MA, Ceccarelli A, Falini A, et al. Brain gray matter changes in migraine patients with T2-visible lesions: a 3-T MRI study. *Stroke.* 2006;37(7):1765–1770.

52. Schmidt-Wilcke T, Gansbauer S, Neuner T, Bogdahn U, May A. Subtle grey matter changes between migraine patients and healthy controls. *Cephalalgia.* 2008;28(1):1–4.

53. Valfre W, Rainero I, Bergui M, Pinessi L. Voxel-based morphometry reveals gray matter abnormalities in migraine. *Headache.* 2008;48(1):109–117.

54. Schmidt-Wilcke T, Leinisch E, Straube A, et al. Gray matter decrease in patients with chronic tension type headache. *Neurology.* 2005;65(9):1483–1486.

55. Apkarian AV, Sosa Y, Sonty S, et al. Chronic back pain is associated with decreased prefrontal and thalamic gray matter density. *J Neurosci.* 2004;24(46):10410–10415.

56. Draganski B, Moser T, Lummel N, et al. Decrease of thalamic gray matter following limb amputation. *Neuroimage.* 2006;31(3):951–957.

57. Kuchinad A, Schweinhardt P, Seminowicz DA, Wood PB, Chizh BA, Bushnell MC. Accelerated brain gray matter loss in fibromyalgia patients: premature aging of the brain?. *J Neurosci.* 2007;27(15):4004–4007.

58. Schmidt-Wilcke T, Luerding R, Weigand T, et al. Striatal grey matter increase in patients suffering from fibromyalgia—a voxel-based morphometry study. *Pain.* 2007;132(suppl 1):S109–S116.

59. Blankstein U, Chen J, Diamant NE, Davis KD. Altered brain structure in irritable bowel syndrome: potential contributions of pre-existing and disease-driven factors. *Gastroenterology.* 2010;138(5):1783–1789.

60. Davis KD, Pope G, Chen J, Kwan CL, Crawley AP, Diamant NE. Cortical thinning in IBS: implications for homeostatic, attention, and pain processing. *Neurology.* 2008;70(2):153–154.

61. Geha PY, Baliki MN, Harden RN, Bauer WR, Parrish TB, Apkarian AV. The brain in chronic CRPS pain: abnormal gray-white matter interactions in emotional and autonomic regions. *Neuron.* 2008;60(4):570–581.

62. Valet M, Gundel H, Sprenger T, et al. Patients with pain disorder show gray-matter loss in pain-processing structures: a voxel-based morphometric study. *Psychosom Med.* 2009;71(1):49–56.

63. As-Sanie S, Harris RE, Napadow V, et al. Changes in regional gray matter volume in women with chronic pelvic pain: a voxel-based morphometry study. *Pain.* 2012;153(5):1006–1014.

64. 1.5.1 Chronic Migraine. *IHS Classification ICHD-II* [Web]. <http://ihs-classification. org/en/02_klassifikation/02_teil1/01.05.01_migraine.html>; 2012.

65. Matharu MS, Good CD, May A, Bahra A, Goadsby PJ. No change in the structure of the brain in migraine: a voxel-based morphometric study. *Eur J Neurol.* 2003;10(1):53–57.

66. DaSilva AF, Granziera C, Snyder J, Hadjikhani N. Thickening in the somatosensory cortex of patients with migraine. *Neurology.* 2007;69(21):1990–1995.

67. Kopf A. Chapter 27: chronic nonspecific back pain. In: Olaogun MOB, ed. *Guide to Pain Management in Low-Resource Settings.* Seattle: International Association for the Study of PAIN; 2010. p. 207–212.

68. Schmidt-Wilcke T, Leinisch E, Gansssbauer S, et al. Affective components and intensity of pain correlate with structural differences in gray matter in chronic back pain patients. *Pain.* 2006;125(1-2):89–97.

69. Elbert T, Flor H, Birbaumer N, et al. Extensive reorganization of the somatosensory cortex in adult humans after nervous system injury. *Neuroreport.* 1994;5(18):2593–2597.

70. Flor H, Elbert T, Knecht S, et al. Phantom-limb pain as a perceptual correlate of cortical reorganization following arm amputation. *Nature.* 1995;375(6531):482–484.

71. Florence SL, Taub HB, Kaas JH. Large-scale sprouting of cortical connections after peripheral injury in adult macaque monkeys. *Science.* 1998;282(5391):1117–1121.

72. Grusser SM, Winter C, Muhlnickel W, et al. The relationship of perceptual phenomena and cortical reorganization in upper extremity amputees. *Neuroscience.* 2001;102(2):263–272.

73. Complex Regional Pain Syndrome. *Mayo Clinic: Diseases and Conditions.* <http://www.mayoclinic.com/health/complex-regional-pain-syndrome/DS00265/ DSECTION=causes>; 2011.

74. *Diagnostic and Statistical Manual of Mental Disorders.* 4th ed. American Psychiatric Association; 2000.

75. Schaeffer AJ, Datta NS, Fowler Jr JE, et al. Overview summary statement. Diagnosis and management of chronic prostatitis/chronic pelvic pain syndrome (CP/CPPS). *Urology.* 2002;60(6 suppl):1–4.

76. Farmer MA, Chanda ML, Parks EL, Baliki MN, Apkarian AV, Schaeffer AJ. Brain functional and anatomical changes in chronic prostatitis/chronic pelvic pain syndrome. *J Urol.* 2011;186(1):117–124.

77. Schweinhardt P, Kuchinad A, Pukall CF, Bushnell MC. Increased gray matter density in young women with chronic vulvar pain. *Pain.* 2008;140(3):411–419.

78. Baliki MN, Geha PY, Apkarian AV, Chialvo DR. Beyond feeling: chronic pain hurts the brain, disrupting the default-mode network dynamics. *J Neurosci.* 2008;28(6):1398–1403.

79. Seminowicz DA, Wideman TH, Naso L, et al. Effective treatment of chronic low back pain in humans reverses abnormal brain anatomy and function. *J Neurosci.* 2011;31(20):7540–7550.

80. Young IR, Randell CP, Kaplan PW, James A, Bydder GM, Steiner RE. Nuclear magnetic resonance (NMR) imaging in white matter disease of the brain using spin-echo sequences. *J Comput Assist Tomogr.* 1983;7(2):290–294.

81. Goto K, Ishii N, Fukasawa H. Diffuse white-matter disease in the geriatric population. A clinical, neuropathological, and CT study. *Radiology.* 1981;141(3):687–695.

82. Rose SE, Chen F, Chalk JB, et al. Loss of connectivity in Alzheimer's disease: an evaluation of white matter tract integrity with colour coded MR diffusion tensor imaging. *J Neurol Neurosurg Psychiatr.* 2000;69(4):528–530.

83. Bozzali M, Falini A, Franceschi M, et al. White matter damage in Alzheimer's disease assessed *in vivo* using diffusion tensor magnetic resonance imaging. *J Neurol Neurosurg Psychiatr*. 2002;72(6):742–746.
84. Scheltens P, Barkhof F, Valk J, et al. White matter lesions on magnetic resonance imaging in clinically diagnosed Alzheimer's disease. Evidence for heterogeneity. *Brain*. 1992;115(Pt 3):735–748.
85. O'Brien J, Desmond P, Ames D, Schweitzer I, Harrigan S, Tress B. A magnetic resonance imaging study of white matter lesions in depression and Alzheimer's disease. *Br J Psychiatr*. 1996;168(4):477–485.
86. Brant-Zawadzki M, Fein G, Van Dyke C, Kiernan R, Davenport L, de Groot J. MR imaging of the aging brain: patchy white-matter lesions and dementia. *AJNR Am J Neuroradiol*. 1985;6(5):675–682.
87. Barber R, Scheltens P, Gholkar A, et al. White matter lesions on magnetic resonance imaging in dementia with Lewy bodies, Alzheimer's disease, vascular dementia, and normal aging. *J Neurol Neurosurg Psychiatr*. 1999;67(1):66–72.
88. Kutzelnigg A, Lucchinetti CF, Stadelmann C, et al. Cortical demyelination and diffuse white matter injury in multiple sclerosis. *Brain*. 2005;128(Pt 11):2705–2712.
89. Loevner LA, Grossman RI, Cohen JA, Lexa FJ, Kessler D, Kolson DL. Microscopic disease in normal-appearing white matter on conventional MR images in patients with multiple sclerosis: assessment with magnetization-transfer measurements. *Radiology*. 1995;196(2):511–515.
90. Lim KO, Hedehus M, Moseley M, de Crespigny A, Sullivan EV, Pfefferbaum A. Compromised white matter tract integrity in schizophrenia inferred from diffusion tensor imaging. *Arch Gen Psychiatr*. 1999;56(4):367–374.
91. Szabo N, Kincses ZT, Pardutz A, et al. White matter microstructural alterations in migraine: a diffusion-weighted MRI study. *Pain*. 2012;153(3):651–656.
92. Chen JY, Blankstein U, Diamant NE, Davis KD. White matter abnormalities in irritable bowel syndrome and relation to individual factors. *Brain Res*. 2011;1392:121–131.
93. Rodriguez-Raecke R, Niemeier A, Ihle K, Ruether W, May A. Brain gray matter decrease in chronic pain is the consequence and not the cause of pain. *J Neurosci*. 2009;29(44):13746–13750.
94. Maleki N, Becerra L, Brawn J, Bigal M, Burstein R, Borsook D. Concurrent functional and structural cortical alterations in migraine. *Cephalalgia*. 2012;32(8):607–620.
95. May A, Ashburner J, Buchel C, et al. Correlation between structural and functional changes in brain in an idiopathic headache syndrome. *Nat Med*. 1999;5(7):836–838.
96. DaSilva AF, Becerra L, Pendse G, Chizh B, Tully S, Borsook D. Colocalized structural and functional changes in the cortex of patients with trigeminal neuropathic pain. *PLoS One*. 2008;3(10):e3396.
97. Baliki MN, Petre B, Torbey S, et al. Corticostriatal functional connectivity predicts transition to chronic back pain. *Nat Neurosci*. 2012;Jul(1)
98. Upadhyay J, Maleki N, Potter J, et al. Alterations in brain structure and functional connectivity in prescription opioid-dependent patients. *Brain*. 2010;133(Pt 7):2098–2114.
99. Maleki N, Linnman C, Brawn J, Burstein R, Becerra L, Borsook D. Her versus his migraine: multiple sex differences in brain function and structure. *Brain*. 2012;135(Pt 8):2546–2559.

Thalamic Burst Firing in Response to Experimental Pain Stimuli and in Patients with Chronic Neuropathic Pain may be a Carrier for Pain-Related Signals

T.M. Markman[1], C.C. Liu[1], J.C. Zhang[1], K. Kobayashi[2], J.H. Kim[3] and F.A. Lenz[1]

[1]Department of Neurosurgery, Johns Hopkins University, Baltimore, Maryland, USA, [2]Department of Neurological Surgery, Division of Applied Systems Neuroscience, and Department of Advanced Medical Science, Nihon University, Tokyo, Japan, [3]Department of Neurosurgery, Ansan Hospital, Korea University, Soeul, Korea

INTRODUCTION

Over the past three decades, functional imaging studies have resulted in substantial progress in our understanding of pain mechanisms in the forebrain.[1] As a result of these imaging studies, pain is viewed as a complex experience that is associated with increased blood flow or BOLD signals in multiple structures in the brain,[2–6] which has been characterized as a "network" or "neuro-matrix,"[7–11] rather than as a collection of unrelated centers,[12] each subserving a different dimension of pain.[12] The pain network includes cortical modules such as medial frontal cortex, MF including middle cingulate cortex (MCC), and supplementary motor area (SMA), primary sensory cortex (SI), and parasylvian cortex (PS including opercular and insular cortex).[3,4,6,11]

A network consists of a collection of neural elements, their connections, and connectional weights, often equated with neurons or brain modules, axons, and synapses, respectively.[13] The functional connectivity of such a network may be conceived of as the network properties that enable its neural elements jointly to process inputs or outputs, or both. We will focus on activity in the principal somatic sensory nucleus, Ventral caudal (Vc) of the thalamus and the SI cortex, which receives dense projection from Vc. The first priority of this review is to consider the evidence that SI and Vc is involved in pain processing. We will then describe pain related abnormalities in Vc and SI.

PAIN-RELATED ACTIVITY IN SI CORTEX

Imaging studies are an important line of evidence of structures involved in the processing of pain. Painful stimuli may produce increased blood flow positron emission tomography (PET) and increased BOLD signals in contralateral human SI.[1,9,14–22] Other studies have failed to find pain-related activity in SI using PET.[23–28] Failure to identify pain-related activity in SI has also been reported in studies of potentials evoked by painful stimuli and recorded using magneto-encephalographic (MEG) and EEG techniques.[29–34] The lack of activation of SI may be related to cognitive factors (e.g. distraction), failure to resolve small somatotopically appropriate activations in SI, and mixed inhibitory/excitatory effects within cortex.[21]

Studies of anesthetized monkeys[35–37] and human MEG studies[37–39] suggest that these pain related effects may result from activation of subunits within SI including area 3a,[37] of area 1,[38,40] or at the border between areas 1 and 3b.[36] A recent anatomical study has identified projections from putative nociceptive, thalamic nucleus ventral medial posterior (VMpo) to BA 3a and 1 (see[34] cf.[41]).

Numerous studies have employed microelectrode techniques to identify neurons in SI that respond to painful stimuli in a graded fashion (WDR, wide dynamic range) or a selective fashion (NS, nociceptive specific). These studies demonstrated that populations with WDR and NS response properties to mechanical or thermal stimuli or both were found among single neurons in S1.[36,40,42] S1 neurons with selective responses to noxious tooth pulp stimuli have been reported in awake monkeys.[43]

S1 neurons responsive to noxious stimuli seem to encode the intensity of these stimuli in awake monkeys.[42] This study measured the response to a small increase in temperature (T2) occurring during a larger step of temperature, from adapting temperature into the painful range. The latency of the monkey's response to the different sizes of the smaller temperature step was correlated with the neuronal response of WDR neurons to the same stimuli.

An important strategy to clarify human neuronal mechanisms of pain is the use of a painful cutaneous laser stimulus to activate cutaneous nociceptors selectively,[32,44,45] which leads to laser evoked potentials (LEPs) and changes in EEG power and synchrony. We have used a thulium YAG laser with a laser-beam wavelength of $2\,\mu m$, a beam diameter of 6 mm, and a duration of 1 ms. A series of recent studies have examined LEPs recorded from the cortical surface, during subdural grid implantations for the treatment of epilepsy. When LEPs and ongoing EEG signals are recorded from the scalp, they are limited by muscle and blink artifacts. They are also limited by low pass and spatial filtering by CSF, skull and scalp.

Source analysis of LEP generators in the region of SI demonstrated two LEP sources. The first was a tangential source at approximately the location of the SI generator, consistent with the area 1 subdivision of SI.[46,47] The other was a radial generator deep to the SEP generator and to the crest of the central sulcus, consistent with area 3a. LEPs consist of an early negative (N2) and late positive potential (P2). The P2 peak was associated with polarity reversal over the central sulcus consistent with a generator in SI.

Loss of sensitivity to painful stimuli by quantitative sensory testing (QST) after CNS lesions, which involve structures showing electrical responses to painful stimuli, can identify structures, which are essential for pain sensations. A recent psychophysical study of a patient with a stroke including the S1 and S2 post-central gyrus reported loss of the sensory but not the unpleasantness dimension of pain.[48] A patient with anatomical resection of the postcentral gyrus for treatment of epilepsy demonstrated thermal hypoesthesia and heat hypoalgesia.[49]

The clearest evidence for the effect of S1 lesions on sensation is found in a study of two monkeys before and after anatomic lesions of S1.[50] Pain detection was measured using the paradigm requiring detection of small temperature steps occurring on a larger temperature step (T1) into the noxious range. Detection of the smaller temperature changes in the noxious range is analogous to detection of pain. The magnitude of the decreased detection tended toward, but did not reach, preoperative levels over a three month period. In order to control for cognitive effects, such as attention or grading performance, the protocol included a visual control. The protocol consisted of a discrimination of light intensity, which changed with steps analogous to the T1 and T2 steps. The lesions had no effect on the performance of the visual task. Together clinical studies and experimental studies in monkeys are strong evidence for the role of S1 cortex in pain detection.

CORTICAL PAIN NETWORK

Our studies of pain-related causality have demonstrated that attention to a painful stimulus leads to a consistent increase in directed functional interactions in pain-related cortical modules during both the pre-stimulus and post-stimulus periods. Directed functional interactions between these structures were calculated by a method (event-related causality, ERC) based on Granger causality.[51–53] Causality is a property by which the signal at one electrode exerts a causal influence upon the signal at another electrode. The technique of ERC has now been applied to signals recorded from grids of electrodes implanted over the cortex during the surgical treatment of epilepsy.[53,54]

Analysis of causality based on signals recorded from cortical electrodes can provide a high resolution picture of the direction and magnitude of interactions in the pain network. SI consistently had significantly more ERC interactions upon PS during the attention task versus the distraction task in the pre-stimulus period.[53] During the post-stimulus period, SI had significant ERC interactions upon PS and MF during the attention task. During both the pre-stimulus and post-stimulus period, there were more "within-area" significant ERC pairs during attention than distraction for SI, but not for PS and MF. This "within-area" ERC may be the result of a local network organized on the basis of neuronal response properties, as in the case of other primary sensory cortical areas.[55] These directed functional interactions between cortical electrode sites may be the result of interactions between cortical sites or indirect interactions through unobserved sites, such as the thalamus.

Some kinds of cortical activity clearly reflect cortical processing of thalamic inputs. For example, spatial attention evokes neuronal activity in Brodmann area 7B, which is a part of PS.[56] Thalamic activity may drive synchronous cortical activity through thalamic oscillations, or through common inputs from the spinothalamic tract (STT) to the thalamic somatic sensory relay nuclear complex to SI.[57–59] SI shows stimulus-evoked responses which increase across the intensive continuum into the painful range (analog functions), while SII may show responses which increase with the stimulus, but only for stimuli in the painful range (binary functions).[60,61] A similar dichotomy of stimulus-response functions has been observed in electrophysiological studies of the thalamic nuclei projecting to SI and SII.[62,63] Therefore, the combination of thalamic modules and cortical "within-area" and "between area." ERC pairs may produce the distinct functions which characterize these human cortical modules.

While there are significant limitations to studies in humans, these studies also provide definite technical advantages, particularly in the resolution of signals recorded from the human brain. For example, recordings directly from the human brain have the unprecedented temporal and spatial resolution of thalamic neuronal spike trains (500 Hz, <0.3 mm), and recordings of multiple neurons (multi-unit recording and local field potentials, LFPs) in the cortex (200 Hz, <1 cm,[53]), and the thalamus (200 Hz, 2–3 mm[4]). These approaches represent a significant technical advantage in the study of human pain-related networks, which currently include PET (<1 Hz, >1 cm), fMRI (10 Hz, <1 cm), and scalp EEG (scalp EEG 80 Hz, >5 cm).[4] The temporal resolution of these human recordings supports the LFP studies of ERC, and the spatial resolution supports the interpretation of the results in terms of the literature of basic neuroscience.

PAIN PROCESSING IN THE REGION OF VC

The human principal sensory nucleus (Vc)[64] is divided into a core area (equivalent to monkey VP, see[65,66]), posterior and inferior regions. These two regions are defined relative to the most posterior and inferior cell with a response to non-painful, cutaneous stimuli. In the core, the majority of cells respond to innocuous, mechanical, cutaneous stimulation. As shown in Figure 3.2, this latter area corresponds to the posterior and inferior subnuclei of Vc which are ventral caudal portae (Vcpor), ventral caudal parvocellular nucleus, (Vcpc),[67] the posterior nucleus, and the magnocellular medial geniculate.[67–69] Studies of patients at autopsy following lesions of the STT show terminations in all these nuclei.[67,70,71] This area includes the ventral medial nucleus—posterior part (VMpo) that may receive STT inputs and may signal pain and temperature ([34,72] cf.[41,73]). The physiology recapitulates this anatomy.

Cells in Vc responding to painful and thermal stimuli are of several types, including WDR and NS cells responding to painful thermal and mechanical stimuli.[63] Some low threshold cells respond to non-painful mechanical and cold stimuli.[63,74,75] Cells in the core and posterior region respond only to noxious heat stimuli[62,75] and to noxious cold stimuli.[76]

Nociceptive cells in Vc appear to signal pain based on lesioning and stimulation studies. Temporary disruption of the activity in the region of Vc has been carried out by injection of local anesthetic into monkey VP, corresponding to human Vc.[66] These injections significantly interfere with the monkey's ability to discriminate temperature in both the innocuous and noxious range.[77] Permanent disruption of activity in this region has been studied in patients with very small thalamic strokes. In this study, impaired discrimination of tactile sensation, cold, or cold pain sensations occurred only in larger lesions. This volume-dependent impairment of sensations may be related to the monkey's anatomical[78–80] and human psychophysical subnuclear divisions of modality specificity within Vc.[78–80] These elements may also be the basis of separate, subnuclear thalamic networks for painful and non-painful modalities.[81]

Another line of evidence for pain processing in the region of Vc is that stimulation within Vc and the regions posterior and inferior to it can evoke the sensations of pain[69,82–84] and temperature.[69,76] The largest study of stimulation-evoked pain and temperature responses examined results of threshold microstimulation of the region of Vc in 124 thalami (116 patients). The location of pain and temperature responses is defined relative to the posterior and inferior borders of Vc. Warm sensations were evoked more frequently in the posterior region (5.7%) than in the core (2.3%). Otherwise the proportions were not significantly different for cool or pain sensations between the core or the posterior region or both (cool 2.5%, 2.2%; pain 2.8%, 4.1%). Warm sensations were evoked more frequently in the lateral plane (10.8%) than in the medial planes of the posterior region (3.9%) but no other significant medial lateral differences for any sensation were found in the core or posterior region or overall.

These more recent results are in contrast to previous studies reporting that a larger proportion of thermal/pain sites were evoked in the posterior and inferior regions.[69,85] These latter studies took a radiological landmark of the thalamus (anterior commissure-posterior commissure line, ACPC) as the floor of Vc, contrary to atlas and physiological maps.[86,87] The more recent study suggests that sites where thermal or pain sensations are evoked are located both within and posterior, inferior, and medial to Vc.

In summary, the evidence of thalamic STT terminations of the pain-related neuronal activity and of microstimulation-evoked sensations suggests that the region is involved in pain processing. Finally the studies of lesions demonstrated that this region is essential for some components of tactile, thermal and of pain processing.

THALAMIC BURST FIRING PATTERNS

An important component of thalamic activity is the low threshold spike (LTS); a calcium conductance which is inactivated at resting membrane potentials but is deinactivated by membrane hyperpolarization.[88] The LTS burst consists of a characteristic train of action potentials, which follow an inhibitory event, manifest by a silent period in the spike train (Figure 3.1). The resolution of thalamic neuronal recordings is high enough to predict the occurrence of membrane events such as bursts of action potentials which result from a membrane low threshold spike (LTS), a calcium conductance.[89,90]

The LTS bursts which follow an inhibitory event have long been associated with behavioral states such as slow wave sleep.[91–93] More recent reports demonstrate that LTS bursts occur during wakefulness in humans[94–96] and in monkeys.[97–98] In addition to the association between LTS bursting and state, there is now evidence that thalamic LTS bursting rates can increase from baseline during sensory stimuli or motor events.[99–103] In monkeys, thalamic LTS bursts occur in neurons in the lateral geniculate nucleus following microscopic eye movements (microsaccades) which occur during visual fixation.[102] This activity must be transmitted to V1 cortex where bursts of action potentials are likewise related to microsaccades and to visual stimuli.[102,104]

LTS bursting increases the synaptic efficacy of thalamo-cortical transmission related to somatic sensation[105] and so may influence sensory psychophysics. We now review evidence that LTS burst firing is related to cognitive tasks, to experimental pain stimuli, and to neuropathic pain defined as "pain arising as a direct consequence of a lesion or disease affecting the somatosensory system".[106]

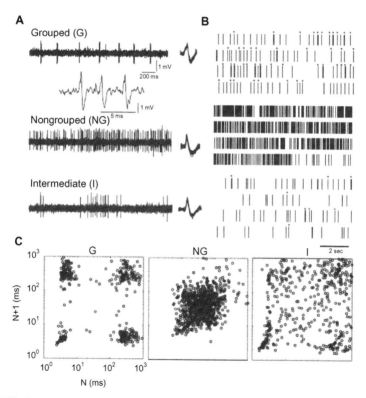

FIGURE 3.1 **A** shows spike trains for three different categories of firing patterns. **B** shows rasters and **C** shows n versus n + 1 plots for these categories as labeled. See text. *Adapted from,[125] with permission.*

THALAMIC FIRING PATTERNS IN RELATION-DIRECTED ATTENTION AND DISTRACTION

We have recently examined firing and LTS burst characteristics during a cognitive task, which involves quiet wakefulness (spontaneous condition) versus mental arithmetic (counting condition). Recordings in the region of Vc were carried out during the awake stereotactic procedures for the treatment of tremor using high impedance microelectrodes and analysis of single neurons by standard techniques.[107,108] Across all neurons and epochs, pre-burst interspike intervals (PBISIs) were bimodal at median values consistent with the duration of GABAa (gamma amino butyric acid subtype a) and GABAb IPSPs (inhibitory postsynaptic potentials). Neuronal spike trains (117 neurons) were categorized by their interspike interval distributions into those firing as LTS bursts (G, grouped), firing as single spikes (NG, non-grouped), or firing as single spikes with sporadic LTS bursting (I, intermediate).

An LTS burst composed of three action potentials is shown in the inset of Figure 3.1A upper (G category). Note that the interspike intervals (ISIs) between these action potentials are very short, approximately 3.5 ms. Dots above the raster in Figure 3.1B indicate the occurrence of LTS bursts of this type. Figure 3.1C shows the n versus n + 1 plot for the three categories, a bias free technique for measuring neuronal LTS bursting activity. These plots are produced by graphing the ISI before an action potential in a spike train (n) versus the ISI after that action potential (n + 1) (Figure 3.1C).

These n versus n + 1 plots provide a graphical display of the characteristics of the spike train overall as reflected by clusters of points in the plot. In the plots of n versus n + 1, the cluster at the lower right indicates a long ISI (approximately 200 to 1000 ms, see Figure 3.1B left) followed by a short ISI (< 6 ms), the defining characteristic of the first spike in an LTS burst, which is post-inhibitory. The lower left and upper right clusters indicate the ISIs within and between bursts, respectively.

Spike trains in the NG category showed high frequency spontaneous firing during the spike train (Figure 3.1B middle) resulting in n versus n + 1 plots characterized by a central cluster and by the absence of clusters at the four corners of the n versus n + 1 plot. Particularly the cluster in the lower right is not seen which is the characteristic post-inhibitory short ISI seen in G spike trains.

Spike trains in the intermediate (I) category had irregular spike firing and common LTS bursts (Figure 3.1A bottom). The clusters in the I category are consistent with the lower right and lower left clusters of the G category (B, left). In addition, the I category of spike trains usually has a central cluster similar to that seen in the NG category.

Our recent studies show that ratios of the numbers of spike trains responding to the painful laser/numbers of spike trains occur preferentially in I category spike trains versus the NG and G firing patterns, based on recordings in 7 subjects (11/12 vs 1/8, P = 0.0008, Fisher). These studies do not determine the relationship of this thalamic activity to activity in cerebral cortex, specifically LEPs and EEG activity in response to a painful laser stimulus. Neither do they establish whether this activity is related to pain-related cognitive tasks or is specific to painful versus non-painful stimuli.

To assess the effect of cognitive task, the activity of thalamic neurons was measured during quiet waking with eyes open (spontaneous condition) versus mental arithmetic in which subjects repeatedly subtracted 7 from 100 (counting condition). During the spontaneous condition (46 neurons), only I spike trains changed category. Overall, burst rates (BR) were lower and firing rates (FR) were higher during the counting versus the spontaneous condition. Spike trains in the G category sometimes changed to I and NG categories at the transition to the counting condition, while those in the I category often changed to NG.

Among spike trains that did not change category by condition, G spike trains had lower BRs during counting, while NG spike trains had higher FRs. BRs were significantly greater than zero for G and I categories during wakefulness (both conditions). The changes between the spontaneous and counting conditions are most pronounced for the I category, which may be a mechanism for event- and cognitive-related changes in CNS activity.

Spike trains in the I category frequently changed category during the spontaneous period, and were composed of both single spikes and LTS bursts, unlike the G and NG category spike trains. These characteristics of the I category are compatible with high variability of membrane conductance, as suggested by modeling studies and studies of a thalamic slice.[109,110] These proposed changes in conductance could result from cortico-thalamic connections, which provide a dense excitatory input both to the distal dendrites of thalamocortical neurons, and to the inhibitory interneurons projecting to thalamocortical neurons.[111–114]

During the spontaneous condition and at the transition to the counting condition, spike trains in the I category have a significantly greater propensity to change categories than the G and NG categories. Overall, these changes suggest that the I category may be a transitional firing pattern between the thalamic burst mode (G category) and the relay mode (NG).

THALAMIC FIRING PATTERNS IN RELATION TO PAINFUL STIMULI

Bursting activity was also measured in neurons categorized by their response to temperature stimuli in the non-painful and painful range. All neuronal categories had clear stimulus-evoked LTS bursting as identified by the criteria for selecting bursts in the spike train as above. Significant pre-burst inhibition is indicated by PBISI not significantly less than 100ms. All neurons responding to pain and non-painful temperature stimuli showed stimulus–evoked bursting composed of small numbers of action potentials.

These PBISI results suggest that the rate of stimulus-evoked LTS burst-ing is dependent upon the rate of inhibitory events. The analysis of LTS burst parameters indicates that the inhibitory circuitry mediating LTS bursting is similar among neuronal types so that LTS bursting influences the activity of all thalamic cell types encoding of pain and temperature. These results do not prove that burst firing is related to pain and tem-perature sensation. This relationship is supported by studies of the sensa-tions evoked by different patterns of stimuli of thalamic microstimulation.

Microstimulation in the region of Vc with patterns similar to LTS burst-ing often evokes sensations like those produced by the somatic sensory stimuli, which produce the same sensations. Specifically, the threshold current at 300Hz was applied at five frequencies (10, 20, 38, 100, and 200Hz) in bursts of 4, 7, 20, 50, and 100 pulses in an ascending stair-case protocol.[62] This is a protocol that is commonly used in studies of pain,[115,116] including our prior studies.[117] This protocol resulted in a facto-rial delivery of all pairs (steps on the staircase) of five frequencies and five numbers of pulses. The results demonstrated that thermal and pain sensa-tions were often evoked 4 or 7 pulses at high frequencies, which is consis-tent with ISI characteristics of LTS.[80] The relationship of LTS bursting to pain is also evident in the thalamic response to the painful laser stimulus.

Thalamic neuronal responses to the painful cutaneous laser demon-strate that many thalamic neurons respond to the laser with early and/or late latency peaks of activity. These latencies are also consistent with conduction of the response to the laser stimulus through pathways from Aδ and C fibers to the thalamus. The responses of these thalamic neurons to the laser stimulus sometimes included LTS bursts of action potentials, consistent with studies reviewed above. Spike trains of laser responsive neurons were more common in the I category, while those of laser non-responsive neurons were more common in the NG category. Therefore, neuronal spike trains in the I category may be a carrier of pain signals to cortex and so mediate the effects of attention to painful stimuli.

THALAMIC FIRING PATTERNS IN CHRONIC PAIN

Thalamic neuronal activity was recorded during procedures to implant electrodes in the thalamus for the treatment of chronic pain secondary to spinal cord injury or amputation. Activity was also recorded in patients with essential tremor and no abnormality of the somatic sensory system during intervals without tremor.

Figure 3.2 shows an example of recordings and responses to stimulation in the thalamus of a patient with neuropathic pain following a T8 spinal cord transaction.[118] In the 15 mm lateral plane (Figure 3.2A, upper) the receptive fields (RFs) and projected fields were all referred to the hand, a part of the representational homunculus, which is above the level of the transaction. The next trajectory (Figure 3.2B upper) was in the

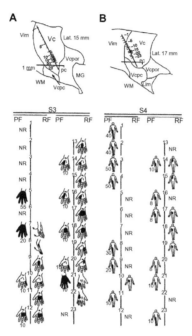

FIGURE 3.2   **Maps of receptive fields (RFs) and projected fields for trajectories in the region of the principal sensory nucleus of the thalamus (Vc) in a patient with spinal cord transection at thoracic level 8. A:** Trajectory in the 15 mm lateral parasagittal plane (Lat 15 mm) through the region of Vc that represents the arm. **B:** trajectory 2 mm lateral to the 1 st (Lat 17 mm). Top panels in **A** and **B:** position of the trajectory relative to nuclear boundaries as predicted radiologically. The anterior commissure (AC)-posterior commissure (PC) line is indicated by the horizontal line in the panel, whereas the trajectories are shown by the oblique lines. Ticks at right of trajectory: locations of cells. Long ticks: cells with RFs. Short ticks: cells without RFs. Stimulation sites are shown at left of the trajectory. Long ticks: Somatosensory response to stimulation. Short ticks: No response to stimulation. The "region of Vc" includes sites 7–23 in A and sites 9–23 in B. Scales are as indicated. The position of nuclei is inferred from the AC–PC line and so is only an approximation of nuclear location. Abbreviations: Vcpor, ventralis caudalis portae; Vcpc, ventralis caudalis parvocellularis; Lim, limitans; MG, medial geniculate; WM, white matter below the ventral nuclear group; Vim, nucleus ventralis intermedius. Bottom panels in A and B: paired figures for sites as numbered in the middle panel. Figurine at right: RF. NR: cell without RF. Figurine at left: PF for threshold microstimulation (TMS) at that site. Number below figure: threshold (microamperes). At all sites along both trajectories where sensations were evoked, that sensation was described as tingling. *Adapted from,*[118] *with permission.*

17 mm lateral plane, where the representation of the leg is usually found, relative to the hand representation.[87]

In this plane input from the periphery was interrupted by a traumatic spinal cord lesion. Along this trajectory many cells did not have RFs. Those that did have RFs had RFs on the chest wall. This is a larger representation of the chest wall than normal where it usually forms a sliver above the large representation of the extremities. The neurons with chest wall RFs were located at sites where microstimulation-evoked sensations located in the anesthetic lower extremities. Therefore, activity at the borderzone of the sensory loss may be referred to lower extremity, which is consistent with clinical and QST studies of SCI central pain.[119]

In the case of patients with spinal cord injury, the part of the thalamus representing the painful area at and below the level of the spinal cord injury (Figure 3.2B upper) was identified by electrophysiological activity (Figure 3.2B lower).[118] In particular, the activity of neurons in this area was characterized by the absence of cells with RFs and the presence of thalamic microstimulation evoked sensations (Projected Fields, PFs) in the anesthetic part of the body.

In describing the spike train, we have determined the firing rate, the burst rate, and the pre-burst interspike interval, as in previous studies.[103,118,120] The primary event rate was calculated by including all spikes occurring outside bursts plus the first spike in each burst. Therefore, the primary event rate is a measure of the rate of spikes occurring between bursts.[91,121] The pre-burst ISI was interpreted as an inhibitory event, which can indicate the type of GABAergic conductance. We have repeatedly validated, illustrated and published these techniques and these burst criteria in our prior studies.[103,118,120]

In these subjects, most neurons located in the part of the region of Vc representing the anesthetic part of the body were in the I category as characterized by burst firing rates which were 10 X greater than control (see Table 3 in Reference[118]). Single spike firing rates between bursts were not different between control subjects and different thalamic areas representing the parts of the body below and above the spinal transection. In patients with spinal cord transaction, the pre-burst silent periods were 2.6 X greater than in control patients (movement disorders).

In patients with chronic pain following amputations, the region of Vc was divided into those representing the stump or the phantom.[120] Thalamic areas representing the stump were identified by receptive fields and projected fields representing the stump. Areas representing the phantom were identified by the absence of receptive fields and the presence of projected fields on the phantom. In the representation of the stump and phantom, burst rates were 2.5 X greater than control while firing rates were not different and the pre-burst silent period was 2.3 X longer (see Table 1 in Reference[120]).

In patients with neuropathic pain, like that occurring in patients with spinal cord lesions or amputation, the nervous system injury seems to lead to sensitization of the STT-thalamocortical pathway.[122] In such patients, electrical microstimulation in Vc and in the region inferior and posterior to Vc evokes pain sensations more commonly, and non-painful cold less commonly than in patients without neuropathic pain.[95,123] Stimulation of this region evoked pain more commonly in patients with hyperalgesia in the setting of neuropathic pain than in those without hyperalgesia.[69,72,76] Therefore, sensitization of this pathway may lead to the ongoing pain and hyperalgesia of central pain syndromes.

In summary, neurons with the I category firing pattern (Figure 3.1) are more likely to respond to the laser,[124] to change category when the cognitive task changes.[125] Furthermore, I firing pattern is associated with inhibitory events of GABAb duration leading to LTS bursts. This change in inhibitory events, possibly related to GABA receptors, could be the result of anatomical distribution of receptors, or of activity changes in pathways innervating the neuron.[126–129]

I category firing is also more common in the representation of the painful part of the body in the patients with neuropathic pain.[118,120] In this population, pre-burst inhibitions are much longer, perhaps consistent with a GABAb conductance. Therefore, I category firing in thalamic modules may be a gate which enables both the response to the painful laser, and the transmission of that response to the cortex.[105,130]

Thalamic structures are likely modules to interact with the SI module of the pain network based on their involvement in densely inter-connected thalamo-cortical assemblies.[114,131] Cortico-cortical synchrony and GRC may be related to thalamic modules by mechanisms including: divergent pathways, or common input from the thalamus to the cortex, or afferent volleys traversing the thalamus, or intrinsic thalamic oscillations.[132–134]

The neurons with I category firing pattern are more likely to respond to the laser,[124] and to change category when the cognitive task changes.[125] Therefore, I category firing may be a thalamic carrier signal which switches with changes in cognitive task,[125] and so enables both the response to the painful laser,[124] and the transmission of that response to the cortex. Furthermore, the I firing pattern is associated with inhibitory events of GABAb duration leading to LTS bursts, which might be exploited by therapies targeting thalamic GABAergic transmission or LTS channels.[135–137]

Acknowledgements

Some of the studies reviewed in this chapter were supported by the National Institutes of Health—National Institute of Neurological Disorders and Stroke (NS38493 and NS40059 to FAL). None of the authors has conflicts of interest related to this work. We thank L.H. Rowland and J. Winberry for excellent technical assistance.

References

1. Talbot JD, Marrett S, Evans AC, Meyer E, Bushnell MC, Duncan GH. Multiple representations of pain in human cerebral cortex. *Science*. 1991;251:1355–1358.
2. Derbyshire SW. Exploring the pain "neuromatrix". *Curr Rev Pain*. 2000;4:467–477.
3. Apkarian AV, Bushnell MC, Treede R-D, Zubieta JK. Human brain mechanisms of pain perception and regulation in health and disease. *Eur J Pain*. 2005;9:463–484.
4. Lenz FA, Casey KL, Jones EG, Willis Jr WD. *The Human Pain System: Experimental and Clinical Perspectives*, 1st ed. NY: Cambridge University Press; 2010.
5. Rainville P, Bushnell MC, Duncan GH. PET studies of the subjective experience of pain. In: Casey KL, Bushnell MC, eds. *Pain Imaging*. Seattle: IASP Press; 2000. p. 123–156.
6. Davis KD. Studies of pain using functional magnetic resonance imaging. In: Casey KL, Bushnell MC, eds. *Pain Imaging*. Seattle: IASP Press; 2000. p. 195–210.
7. Melzack R. Phantom limbs and the concept of a neuromatrix. *Trends Neurosci*. 1990;13:88–92.
8. Strigo IA, Duncan GH, Boivin M, Bushnell MC. Differentiation of visceral and cutaneous pain in the human brain. *J Neurophysiol*. 2003;89:3294–3303.
9. Gelnar PA, Krauss BR, Sheehe PR, Szeverenyi NM, Apkarian AV. A comparative fMRI study of cortical representations for thermal painful, vibrotactile, and motor performance tasks. *Neuroimage*. 1999;10:460–482.
10. Peyron R, Garcia-Larrea L, Gregoire MC, et al. Haemodynamic brain responses to acute pain in humans: sensory and attentional networks. *Brain*. 1999;122(Pt 9):1765–1780.
11. Casey KL. Concepts of pain mechanisms: the contribution of functional imaging of the human brain. *Prog Brain Res*. 2000;129:277–287.
12. Melzack R, Casey KL. Sensory, motivational, and central control determinants of pain. In: Kenshalo D, ed. *The Skin Senses* (1st ed.). Springfield, Ill: Thomas; 1968. p. 423–443.
13. Churchland PS, Sejnowski TJ. *The Computational Brain*. Cambridge: MIT Press; 1992.
14. Coghill RC, Talbot JD, Evans AC, et al. Distributed processing of pain and vibration by the human brain. *J Neurosci*. 1994;14:4095–4108.
15. Craig AD, Reiman EM, Evans A, Bushnell MC. Functional imaging of an illusion of pain. *Nature*. 1996;384:258–260.
16. Coghill RC, Sang CN, Maisog JM, Iadarola MJ. Pain intensity processing within the human brain: a bilateral, distributed mechanism. *J Neurophysiol*. 1999;82:1934–1943.
17. Ploghaus A, Tracey I, Gati JS, et al. Dissociating pain from its anticipation in the human brain. *Science*. 1999;284:1979–1981.
18. Casey KL, Minoshima S, Berger KL, Koeppe RA, Morrow TJ, Frey KA. Positron emission tomographic analysis of cerebral structures activated specifically by repetitive noxious heat stimuli. *J Neurophysiol*. 1994;71:802–807.
19. Coghill RC, Sang CN, Ma J, Iadarola MJ. Distributed representation of painful stimulus intensity in the human brain [abstract]. Coghill RC, Sang CN, Ma J, Iadarola MJ. *Soc Neurosci Abstr*. 1997;23:439.
20. Derbyshire SWG, Jones AKP, Gyulai F, Clark S, Townsend D, Firestone L. Pain processing during three levels of noxious stimulation produces different pattern of central activity. *Pain*. 1997;73:431–445.
21. Bushnell MC, Duncan GH, Hofbauer RK, Ha B, Chen JI, Carrier B. Pain perception: is there a role for primary somatosensory cortex?. *Proc Natl Acad Sci USA*. 1999;96:7705–7709.
22. Davis KD, Wood ML, Crawley AP, Mikulis DJ. fMRI of human somatosensory and cingulate cortex during painful electrical nerve stimulation. *Neurorep*. 1995;7:321–325.
23. Jones AK, Brown WD, Friston KJ, Qi LY, Frackowiak RS. Cortical and subcortical localization of response to pain in man using positron emission tomography. *Proc R Soc Lond B Biol Sci*. 1991;244:39–44.

24. Derbyshire SW, Jones AK, Devani P, et al. Cerebral responses to pain in patients with atypical facial pain measured by positron emission tomography. *J Neurol Neurosurg Psychiatry*. 1994;57:1166–1172.

25. Rosen SD, Paulesu E, Frith CD, et al. Central nervous pathways mediating angina pectoris. *Lancet*. 1994;344:147–150.

26. Derbyshire SWG, Vogt BA, Jones AKP. Pain and stroop interference tasks activate separate processing modules in anterior cingulate cortex. *Exp Brain Res*. 1998;118:52–60.

27. Hsieh JC, Belfrage M, Stone-Elander S, Hansson P, Ingvar M. Central representation of chronic ongoing neuropathic pain studied by positron emission tomography. *Pain*. 1995;63:225–236.

28. Iadarola MJ, Berman KF, Zeffiro TA, et al. Neural activation during acute capsaicin-evoked pain and allodynia assessed with PET. *Brain*. 1998;121:931–947.

29. Becker DE, Yingling CD, Fein G. Identification of pain, intensity, and P300 components in the pain evoked potential. *EEG Clin Neurophysiol*. 1993;88:290–301.

30. Bench CJ, Frith CD, Grasby PM, Friston KJ, Paulesu E, Frackowiak RSJ. Investigations of the functional anatomy of attention using the stroop test. *Neuropsych*. 1993:907–922.

31. Buchner H, Richrath P, Grunholz J, et al. Differential effects of pain and spatial attention on digit representation in the human primary somatosensory cortex. *Neurorep*. 2000;11:1289–1293.

32. Carmon A, Dotan Y, Sarne Y. Correlation of subjective pain experience with cerebral evoked responses to noxious thermal stimulations. *Exp Brain Res*. 1978;33:445–453.

33. Casey KL, Minoshima S, Morrow TJ, Koeppe RA. Comparison of human cerebral activation pattern during cutaneous warmth, heat pain, and deep cold pain. *J Neurophysiol*. 1996;76:571–581.

34. Craig AD, Bushnell MC, Zhang ET, Blomqvist A. A thalamic nucleus specific for pain and temperature sensation. *Nature*. 1994;372:770–773.

35. Tommerdahl M, Delemos KA, Vierck Jr CJ, Favorov OV, Whitsel BL. Anterior parietal cortical response to tactile and skin-heating stimuli applied to the same skin site. *J Neurophysiol*. 1996;75:2662–2670.

36. Kenshalo Jr DR, Isensee O. Responses of primate SI cortical neurons to noxious stimuli. *J Neurophysiol*. 1983;50:1479–1496.

37. Tommerdahl M, Delemos KA, Favorov OV, Metz CB, Vierck Jr CJ, Whitsel BL. Response of anterior parietal cortex to different modes of same-site skin stimulation. *J Neurophysiol*. 1998;80:3272–3283.

38. Ploner M, Schmitz F, Freund HJ, Schnitzler A. Parallel activation of primary and secondary somatosensory cortices in human pain processing. *J Neurophysiol*. 1999;81:3100–3104.

39. Kanda M, Nagamine T, Ikeda A, et al. Primary somatosensory cortex is actively involved in pain processing in human. *Brain Res*. 2000;853:282–289.

40. Kenshalo DR, Iwata K, Sholas M, Thomas DA. Response properties and organization of nociceptive neurons in area 1 of monkey primary somatosensory cortex. *J Neurophysiol*. 2000;84:719–729.

41. Graziano A, Jones EG. Widespread thalamic terminations of fibers arising in the superficial medullary dorsal horn of monkeys and their relation to calbindin immunoreactivity. *J Neurosci*. 2004;24:248–256.

42. Kenshalo Jr DR, Chudler EH, Anton F, Dubner R. SI nociceptive neurons participate in the encoding process by which monkeys perceive the intensity of noxious thermal stimulation. *Brain Res*. 1988;454:378–382.

43. Chudler EH, Dong WK, Kawakami Y. Cortical nociceptive responses and behavioral correlates in the monkey. *Brain Res*. 1986;397:47–60.

44. Bromm B, Treede RD. Nerve fibre discharges, cerebral potentials and sensations induced by CO_2 laser stimulation. *Hum Neurobiol*. 1984;3:33–40.

45. Carmon A, Mor J, Goldberg J. Evoked cerebral responses to noxious thermal stimuli in humans. *Exp Brain Res.* 1976;25:103–107.
46. Baumgartner U, Vogel H, Ohara S, Treede RD, Lenz FA. Dipole source analyses of early median nerve SEP components obtained from subdural grid recordings. *J Neurophysiol.* 2011;104:3029–3041.
47. Baumgartner U, Vogel H, Ohara S, Treede RD, Lenz FA. Dipole source analyses of laser evoked potentials (LEP) obtained from subdural grid recordings from primary somatic sensory cortex. *J Neurophysiol.* 2011;106:722–730.
48. Ploner M, Freund H-J, Schnitzler A. Pain affect without pain sensation in a patient with a postcentral lesion. *Pain.* 1999;81:211–214.
49. Veldhuijzen DS, Greenspan JD, Kim JH, Lenz FA. Altered pain and thermal sensation in subjects with isolated parietal and insular cortical lesions. *Eur J Pain.* 2009;14 e535-e1–e535-e11.
50. Kenshalo Jr DR, Willis Jr WD. The role of the cerebral cortex in pain sensation. In: Peters A, Jones EG, eds. *Cerebral Cortex, Vol 9 Normal and Altered States of Function* (1st ed.). New York and London: Plenum Press; 1991. p. 153–212.
51. Granger CW. Investigating causal relations by econometric models and cross spectral methods. *Econometri.* 1969;37:424–438.
52. Korzeniewska A, Crainiceanu CM, Kus R, Franaszczuk PJ, Crone NE. Dynamics of event-related causality in brain electrical activity. *Hum Brain Mapp.* 2007
53. Liu CC, Ohara S, Franaszczuk PJ, Lenz FA. Attention to painful cutaneous laser stimuli evokes directed functional connectivity between activity recorded directly from human pain-related cortical structures. *Pain.* 2011;152:664–675.
54. Liu CC, Ohara S, Franaszczuk PJ, Crone NE, Lenz FA. Attention to painful cutaneous laser stimuli evokes directed functional interactions between human sensory and modulatory pain-related cortical areas. *Pain.* 2011;152:2781–2791.
55. Brosch M, Schreiner CE. Correlations between neural discharges are related to receptive field properties in cat primary auditory cortex. *Eur J Neurosci.* 1999;11:3517–3530.
56. Dong WK, Chudler EH, Sugiyama K, Roberts VJ, Hayashi T. Somatosensory, multi-sensory, and task-related neurons in cortical area 7b (PF) of unanesthetized monkeys. *J Neurophysiol.* 1994;72:542–564.
57. Swadlow HA, Beloozerova IN, Sirota MG. Sharp, local synchrony among putative feed-forward inhibitory interneurons of rabbit somatosensory cortex. *J Neurophysiol.* 1998;79:567–582.
58. Swadlow HA. Influence of VPM afferents on putative inhibitory interneurons in S1 of the awake rabbit: evidence from cross-correlation, microstimulation, and latencies to peripheral sensory stimulation. *J Neurophysiol.* 1995;73:1584–1599.
59. Usrey WM, Reid RC. Synchronous activity in the visual system. *Annu Rev Physiol.* 1999;61:435–456.
60. Timmermann L, Ploner M, Haucke K, Schmitz F, Baltissen R, Schnitzler A. Differential coding of pain intensity in the human primary and secondary somatosensory cortex. *J Neurophysiol.* 2001;86:1499–1503.
61. Bornhovd K, Quante M, Glauche V, Bromm B, Weiller C, Buchel C. Painful stimuli evoke different stimulus-response functions in the amygdala, prefrontal, insula and somatosensory cortex: a single-trial fMRI study. *Brain.* 2002;125:1326–1336.
62. Lenz FA, Ohara S, Gracely RH, Dougherty PM, Patel SH. Pain encoding in the human forebrain: binary and analog exteroceptive channels. *J Neurosci.* 2004;24:6540–6544.
63. Lee J, Dougherty PM, Antezana D, Lenz FA. Responses of neurons in the region of human thalamic principal somatic sensory nucleus to mechanical and thermal stimuli graded into the painful range. *J Comp Neurol.* 1999;410:541–555.
64. Hassler R. Anatomy of the thalamus. In: Schaltenbrand G, Bailey P, eds. *Introduction to Stereotaxis with an Atlas of the Human Brain.* Stuttgart: Theime, G.; 1959. p. 230–290.

65. Olszewski J. *The Thalamus of Maccaca Mulatta*. New York: Karger; 1952.
66. Hirai T, Jones EG. A new parcellation of the human thalamus on the basis of histochemical staining. *Brain Res Rev*. 1989;14:1–34.
67. Mehler WR. The posterior thalamic region in man. *Confin Neurol*. 1966;27:18–29.
68. Mehler WR. The anatomy of the so-called "pain tract" in man: an analysis of the course and distribution of the ascending fibers of the fasciculus anterolateralis. In: French JD, Porter RW, eds. *Basic Research in Paraplegia*. Springfield: Thomas; 1962. p. 26–55.
69. Lenz FA, Seike M, Richardson RT, et al. Thermal and pain sensations evoked by microstimulation in the area of human ventrocaudal nucleus. *J Neurophysiol*. 1993;70:200–212.
70. Bowsher D. Termination of the central pain pathway in man: the conscious appreciation of pain. *Brain*. 1957;80:606–620.
71. Mehler WR. Some neurological species differences- A posteriori. *Ann N Y Acad Sci*. 1969;167:424–468.
72. Blomqvist A, Zhang ET, Craig AD. Cytoarchitectonic and immunohistochemical characterization of a specific pain and temperature relay, the posterior portion of the ventral medial nucleus, in the human thalamus. *Brain*. 2000;123(Pt 3):601–619.
73. Willis Jr WD, Zhang X, Honda CN, Giesler Jr GJ. Projections from the marginal zone and deep dorsal horn to the ventrobasal nuclei of the primate thalamus. *Pain*. 2001;92:267–276.
74. Lenz FA, Dougherty PM. Cells in the human principal thalamic sensory nucleus (Ventralis Caudalis—Vc) respond to innocuous mechanical and cool stimuli. *J Neurophysiol*. 1998;79:2227–2230.
75. Lenz FA, Seike M, Lin YC, et al. Neurons in the area of human thalamic nucleus ventralis caudalis respond to painful heat stimuli. *Brain Res*. 1993;623:235–240.
76. Davis KD, Lozano RM, Manduch M, Tasker RR, Kiss ZH, Dostrovsky JO. Thalamic relay site for cold perception in humans. *J Neurophysiol*. 1999;81:1970–1973.
77. Duncan GH, Bushnell MC, Oliveras JL, Bastrash N, Tremblay N. Thalamic VPM nucleus in the behaving monkey. III. Effects of reversible inactivation by lidocaine on thermal and mechanical discrimination. *J Neurophysiol*. 1993;70:2086–2096.
78. Jones EG, Friedman DP, Hendry SH. Thalamic basis of place- and modality-specific columns in monkey somatosensory cortex: a correlative anatomical and physiological study. *J Neurophysiol*. 1982;48:545–568.
79. Rausell E, Bae CS, Vinuela A, Huntley GW, Jones EG. Calbindin and parvalbumin cells in monkey VPL thalamic nucleus: distribution, laminar cortical projections, and relations to spinothalamic terminations. *J Neurosci*. 1992;12:4088–4111.
80. Patel S, Ohara S, Dougherty PM, Gracely RH, Lenz FA. Psychophysical elements of place and modality specificity in the thalamic somatic sensory nucleus (ventral caudal, vc) of awake humans. *J Neurophysiol*. 2006;95:646–659.
81. Apkarian AV, Shi T, Bruggemann J, Airapetian LR. Segregation of nociceptive and non-nociceptive networks in the squirrel monkey somatosensory thalamus. *J Neurophysiol*. 2000;84:484–494.
82. Dostrovsky JO, Wells FEB, Tasker RR. Pain evoked by stimulation in human thalamus. In: Sjigenaga Y, ed. *International Symposium on Processing Nociceptive Information*. Amsterdam: Elsevier; 1991. p. 115–120.
83. Willis WD. *The Pain System*. Basel: Karger; 1985.
84. Hassler R, Reichert T. Klinische und anatomische Befunde bei stereotaktischen Schmerzoperationen im Thalamus. *Arch Psychiat Nerverkr*. 1959;200:93–122.
85. Davis KD, Kiss ZHT, Tasker RR, Dostrovsky JO. Thalamic stimulation-evoked sensations in chronic pain patients and nonpain (movement disorder) patients. *J Neurophysiol*. 1996;75:1026–1037.
86. Schaltenbrand G, Bailey P. *Introduction to Stereotaxis with an Atlas of the Human Brain*. Stuttgart: Thieme; 1959.

87. Lenz FA, Dostrovsky JO, Tasker RR, Yamashiro K, Kwan HC, Murphy JT. Single-unit analysis of the human ventral thalamic nuclear group: somatosensory responses. *J Neurophysiol.* 1988;59:299–316.

88. Jahnsen H, Llinas R. Electrophysiological properties of guinea-pig thalamic neurones: an in vitro study. *J Physiol.* 1984;349:205–226.

89. Sherman SM, Guillery RW. The role of the thalamus in the flow of information to the cortex. *Philos Trans R Soc Lond B Biol Sci.* 2002;357:1695–1708.

90. Livingstone MS, Freeman DC, Hubel DH. Visual responses in V1 of freely viewing monkeys. *Cold Spring Harb Symp Quant Biol.* 1996;61:27–37.

91. McCarley RW, Benoit O, Barrionuevo G. Lateral geniculate nucleus unitary discharge in sleep and waking: state and rate specific aspects. *J Neurophysiol.* 1983;50:798–818.

92. Domich L, Oakson G, Steriade M. Thalamic burst patterns in the naturally sleeping cat: a comparison between cortically-projecting and reticularis neurones. *J Physiol (Lond).* 1986;379:429–449.

93. Steriade M, Jones EG, McCormick DA. Thalamic, organization and chemical neuro-anatomy *Thalamus, Vol. 1.* Amsterdam: Elsevier; 1997. 269–338.

94. Zirh AT, Lenz FA, Reich SG, Dougherty PM. Patterns of bursting occurring in thalamic cells during parkinsonian tremor. *Neurosci.* 1997;83:107–121.

95. Radhakrishnan V, Tsoukatos J, Davis KD, Tasker RR, Lozano AM, Dostrovsky JO. A comparison of the burst activity of lateral thalamic neurons in chronic pain and non-pain patients. *Pain.* 1999;80:567–575.

96. Jeanmonod D, Magnin M, Morel A. Low-threshold calcium spike bursts in the human thalamus. Common physiopathology for sensory, motor and limbic positive symptoms. *Brain.* 1996;119(Pt 2):363–375.

97. Ramcharan EJ, Cox CL, Zhan XJ, Sherman SM, Gnadt JW. Cellular mechanisms underlying activity patterns in the monkey thalamus during visual behavior. *J Neurophysiol.* 2000;84:1982–1987.

98. Ramcharan EJ, Gnadt JW, Sherman SM. Higher-order thalamic relays burst more than first-order relays. *Proc Natl Acad Sci USA.* 2005;102:12236–12241.

99. Ramcharan EJ, Gnadt JW, Sherman SM. State dependent changes in the firing pattern of relay neurons in the monkey LGN. *Soc Neurosci Abstr.* 1998;24:139.

100. Ramcharan EJ, Gnadt JW, Sherman SM. Burst and tonic firing in thalamic cells of unanesthetized, behaving monkeys. *Vis Neurosci.* 2000;17:55–62.

101. Ramcharan EJ, Gnadt JW, Sherman SM. The effects of saccadic eye movements on the activity of geniculate relay neurons in the monkey. *Vis Neurosci.* 2001;18:253–258.

102. Martinez-Conde S, Macknik SL, Hubel DH. The function of bursts of spikes during visual fixation in the awake primate lateral geniculate nucleus and primary visual cortex. *Proc Natl Acad Sci USA.* 2002;99:13920–13925.

103. Lee JI, Ohara S, Dougherty PM, Lenz FA. Pain and temperature encoding in the human thalamic somatic sensory nucleus (Ventral caudal): inhibition-related bursting evoked by somatic stimuli. *J Neurophysiol.* 2005;94:1676–1687.

104. Martinez-Conde S, Macknik SL, Hubel DH. Microsaccadic eye movements and firing of single cells in the striate cortex of macaque monkeys. *Nat Neurosci.* 2000;3:251–258.

105. Swadlow HA, Gusev AG. The impact of "bursting" thalamic impulses at a neocortical synapse. *Nat Neurosci.* 2001;4:402–408.

106. Treede RD, Jensen TS, Campbell JN, et al. Neuropathic pain: redefinition and a grading system for clinical and research purposes. *Neurology.* 2008;70:1630–1635.

107. Lenz FA, Dostrovsky JO, Kwan HC, Tasker RR, Yamashiro K, Murphy JT. Methods for microstimulation and recording of single neurons and evoked potentials in the human central nervous system. *J Neurosurg.* 1988;68:630–634.

108. Kobayashi K, Kim JH, Anderson WS, Lenz FA. Neurosurgical treatment of tremor. In: Winn R, ed. *Youman's Neurological Surgery.* New York: Saunders; 2009. p. 932–937.

109. Wolfart J, Debay D, Le MG, Destexhe A, Bal T. Synaptic background activity controls spike transfer from thalamus to cortex. *Nat Neurosci*. 2005;8:1760–1767.

110. Debay D, Wolfart J, Le FY, Le MG, Bal T. Exploring spike transfer through the thalamus using hybrid artificial-biological neuronal networks. *J Physiol Paris*. 2004;98:540–558.

111. Ahlsen G, Grant K, Lindstrom S. Monosynaptic excitation of principal cells in the lateral geniculate nucleus by corticofugal fibers. *Brain Res*. 1982;234:454–458.

112. Contreras D, Steriade M. Cellular basis of EEG slow rhythms: a study of dynamic corticothalamic relationships. *J Neurosci*. 1995;15:604–622.

113. Liu XB, Honda CN, Jones EG. Distribution of four types of synapse on physiologically identified relay neurons in the ventral posterior thalamic nucleus of the cat. *J Comp Neurol*. 1995;352:69–91.

114. Steriade M, Jones EG, McCormick DA. *Thalamus Organisation and Function*. Amsterdam: Elsevier; 1997.

115. Gracely RH, Lota L, Walter DJ, Dubner R. A multiple random staircase method of psychophysical pain assessment. *Pain*. 1988;32:55–63.

116. Yarnitsky D, Sprecher E. Thermal testing: normative data and repeatability for various test algorithms. *J Neurol Sci*. 1994;125:39–45.

117. Greenspan JD, Ohara S, Sarlani E, Lenz FA. Allodynia in patients with post-stroke central pain (CPSP) studied by statistical quantitative sensory testing within individuals. *Pain*. 2004;109:357–366.

118. Lenz FA, Kwan HC, Martin R, Tasker R, Richardson RT, Dostrovsky JO. Characteristics of somatotopic organization and spontaneous neuronal activity in the region of the thalamic principal sensory nucleus in patients with spinal cord transection. *J Neurophysiol*. 1994;72:1570–1587.

119. Finnerup NB, Johannesen IL, Fuglsang-Frederiksen A, Bach FW, Jensen TS. Sensory function in spinal cord injury patients with and without central pain. *Brain*. 2003;126:57–70.

120. Lenz FA, Garonzik IM, Zirh TA, Dougherty PM. Neuronal activity in the region of the thalamic principal sensory nucleus (ventralis caudalis) in patients with pain following amputations. *Neurosci*. 1998;86:1065–1081.

121. Cox DR, Lewis PAW. *The Statistical Analysis of Series of Events*. London: Chapman and Hall; 1966.

122. Lenz FA, Gracely RH, Baker FH, Richardson RT, Dougherty PM. Reorganization of sensory modalities evoked by microstimulation in region of the thalamic principal sensory nucleus in patients with pain due to nervous system injury. *J Comp Neurol*. 1998;399:125–138.

123. Lenz FA, Byl NN. Reorganization in the cutaneous core of the human thalamic principal somatic sensory nucleus (Ventral caudal) in patients with dystonia. *J Neurophysiol*. 1999;82:3204–3212.

124. Kobayashi K, Winberry J, Liu CC, Treede RD, Lenz FA. A painful cutaneous laser stimulus evokes responses from single neurons in the human thalamic principal somatic sensory nucleus ventral caudal – Vc. *J Neurophysiol*. 2009;101:2210–2217.

125. Kim JH, Ohara S, Lenz FA. Mental arithmetic leads to multiple discrete changes from baseline in the firing patterns of human thalamic neurons. *J Neurophysiol*. 2009;101:2107–2119.

126. Roy JP, Clercq M, Steriade M, Deschenes M. Electrophysiology of neurons of lateral thalamic nuclei in cat: mechanisms of long-lasting hyperpolarizations. *J Neurophysiol*. 1984;51:1220–1235.

127. Soltesz I, Lightowler S, Leresche N, Crunelli V. On the properties and origin of the GABAB inhibitory postsynaptic potential recorded in morphologically identified projection cells of the cat dorsal lateral geniculate nucleus. *Neurosci*. 1989;33:23–33.

128. Sherman SM, Guillery RW. *Exploring the Thalamus and its Role in Cortical Function*, 1st ed. New York: Oxford University Press; 2001.
129. Bal T, von Krosigk M, McCormick DA. Role of the ferret perigeniculate nucleus in the generation of synchronized oscillations in vitro. *J Physiol*. 1995;483(Pt 3):665–685.
130. Swadlow HA, Gusev AG, Bezdudnaya T. Activation of a cortical column by a thalamocortical impulse. *J Neurosci*. 2002;22:7766–7773.
131. Destexhe A, Sejnowski TJ. *Thalamcortical Assemblies*. NY: Oxford University Press; 2001.
132. Burton H. Responses of spinal cord neurons to systematic changes in hindlimb skin temperatures in cats and primates. *J Neurophysiol*. 1975;38:1060–1079.
133. Apkarian AV, Shi T. Squirrel monkey lateral thalamus. I. Somatic nociresponsive neurons and their relation to spinothalamic terminals. *J Neurosci*. 1994;14:6779–6795.
134. Burton H. Corticothalamic connections from the second somatosensory area and neighboring regions in the lateral sulcus of macaque monkeys. *Brain Res*. 1984;309:367–372.
135. Huguenard JR, Prince DA. Intrathalamic rhythmicity studied in vitro: nominal T-current modulation causes robust antioscillatory effects. *J Neurosci*. 1994;14:5485–5502.
136. Porcello DM, Smith SD, Huguenard JR. Actions of U-92032, a T-type Ca2+ channel antagonist, support a functional linkage between I(T) and slow intrathalamic rhythms. *J Neurophysiol*. 2003;89:177–185.
137. Dib-Hajj SD, Cummins TR, Black JA, Waxman SG. Sodium channels in normal and pathological pain. *Annu Rev Neurosci*. 2010;33:325–347.

4

Central Pain: A Thalamic Deafferentation Generating Thalamocortical Dysrhythmia

Rodolfo R. Llinás and Kerry Walton

Dept. of Physiology & Neuroscience, NYU School of Medicine,
New York, USA

INTRODUCTION

The intrinsic electrical properties of neurons are presently considered to be a salient parameter in brain function.[1,2,3,4,5] This is in contrast to the classical purely reflexological view in which neurons are considered to be passive agents that are modulated exclusively by synaptic input. This intrinsic functional view was originally addressed in relation to thalamic neuron function.[6,7] *In vitro* studies showed that thalamic cells have two intrinsic firing patterns, tonic firing when they are at resting potential or depolarized and low frequency bursts when thalamic cells are hyperpolarized.[7] Recurrent thalamocortical loops reinforce these intrinsic patterns.[8,9] Such changes in thalamic firing to a bursting pattern have been associated with central neuropathic pain as well as other disorders.[10,11] They were first recorded from the lateral somatosensory thalamus of patients with neurogenic pain in 1989.[12] From an electrophysiological imaging perspective, EEG[13,14,15] and magnetoencphalography (MEG)[16,17] studies have shown the presence of a distinct increase in low-frequency activation in central pain. In contrast to peripheral pain patients, in addition to somatosensory appropriate low frequency activity, central pain patients have an additional site generating low frequency oscillations in the mesial-orbito frontal and anterior cingulated cortices, as well as the temporal (insular) cortex.[15,16,17] In fact, the presence of low frequency oscillations distinguished between spinal cord injury patients with pain below the level of the lesion from those without such pain[18] and between patients with neuropathic pain and control groups.[14] A decrease in such low frequency oscillations has been associated with pain alleviation.[14,15] Further, central pain can be modulated by peripheral stimulation[19,20] that serves to depolarize thalamic cells switching these cells from a slow phasic to a higher frequency tonic firing pattern.

Direct support for a deafferentation leading to low frequency thalamic firing has been obtained in *in vitro* studies of rodent thalamocortical slices[21] and is an extension of the *in vivo* animal studies concerning neuropathic pain,[22,23] and thalamic deafferentation.[24] These latter results have established a direct relationship between abnormal thalamic rhythmicity and the occurrence of central pain. This view is supported by a rodent *in vivo* study in which allodynia following spinal cord lesion was accompanied by spontaneous oscillatory burst firing of thalamic ventral posterior lateral (VPL) neurons.[22] The abnormal burst responses were maintained for periods as long as 30s in close to 50% of the thalamic cells of allodynic animals, while such activity was absent in control rodents.

Marini et al[25] have identified a delayed, marked increase in cortical theta rhythm and behavioral aberrations following experimentally-induced rostral reticular thalamic lesions. This provides a model of thalamocortical dysrhythmia in awake rats offering a potential model for neuropathic syndromes such as that seen in Dejerine Roussy syndrome.[26]

Here we will address human MEG brain activity recorded from patients with chronic neuropathic pain resulting from input deafferentation (i.e. phantom limb), brachial plexus avulsion, lateral thalamic vascular accident, as well as a group of patients with pain related to peripheral sources.

DEAFFERENTATION PAIN SYNDROMES

Spontaneous brain activity was recorded from three patients with deafferentation pain syndrome (phantom arm, brachial plexus avulsion, lateral thalamic lesion) using MEG.[16]

MEG Power Spectra and Sources of Theta Activity

Spectral analysis in these patients demonstrated distinct power increases in high theta frequency range (7–9 Hz). The spectra were similar to those of other disorders of thalamocortical dysrhythmia (TCD).[10,27] Mean spectral energy in two bands (7–9 Hz and 9–11 Hz) allows

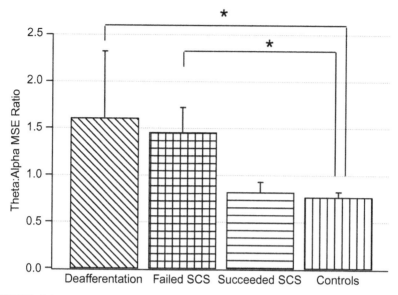

FIGURE 4.1   **Comparisons of mean spectra energy (power ratio 7–9 Hz: 9–11 Hz) in three groups of patients and control group.** Patients in which the SCS did not bring relief (boxes) and those with deafferentation pain (diagonal lines) has significantly more low-frequency activity than the control group (vertical lines) and patients with successful SCS (horizontal lines) The last two groups were not significantly different. (*$p < 0.05$) Subject group comparisons using a Mann-Whitney (unadjusted, one-sided comparison) test found that the control group MSE ratio was significantly different ($p = 0.048$) from the deafferentation group (*modified from Schulman et al.*[16]).

comparison of these results with those of other patient and control groups (Figure 4.1).

Independent component analysis revealed somatotopically meaningful theta-range activity in two of these patients. In the patient with a right thalamus vascular lesion (who suffered from thalamic pain syndrome and tinnitus) theta activity had a right sensorimotor cortex and superior temporal gyrus localization (Figure 4.2). In the patient with a left brachial plexus avulsion theta-range activation localized in the right somatosensory cortex as well as in the temporal and ventromedial frontal cortex.

The limbic source distribution is consistent with reported structural and functional aberrations that have been identified in the context of chronic pain.[28] The finding that limbic sources are present, in parallel with aberrant somatosensory activation underscores the fact that the affective emotional components of the nociceptive experience are physiologically coupled to the specific sensory complaint location.

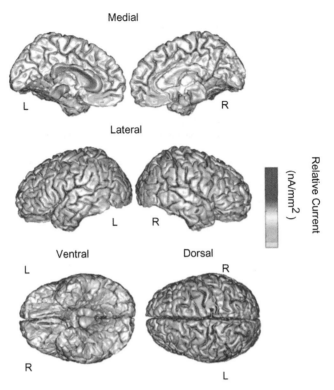

FIGURE 4.2 **Example of localization of theta activity in a patient with brachial plexus avulsion pain.** Activity is localized to the contralateral somatosensory cortex and bilaterally to the mesial orbitofrontal ortices. Scale nA/mm^2 (*modified from Schulman et al.*[16]).

PERIPHERAL PAIN SYNDROMES

In this set of syndromes patients experience chronic pain following well-defined body injuries. Eight such patients had stimulating electrodes implanted in the spinal cord to alleviate the pain. Of these, five reported an over 50% reduction in pain while the other three did not report improvement. MEG recordings were made while the patient's eyes were closed and the spinal cord stimulation (SCS) was turned off.[16]

MEG Power Spectra and Localization

Theta range activity was seen in the power spectra of the three patients who did not receive pain relief with SCS. By contrast, the power spectra from the five patients who obtained relief from SCS were comparable to those of healthy controls.

Independent component localization revealed somatotopically meaningful theta-range activity in two of the patients in the SCS failure group with back pain. There was bilateral theta activation in areas near the classical homunculus sensory representation of the trunk.[29] Comparable independent components were not present in patients with successful SCS or in healthy, pain-free controls.

SCS and Thalamocortical Dysrhythmia

The differences in spectral properties between the failed SCS and successful SCS groups, in addition to the similarity of the former with the deafferentation group, suggests that non-dysrhythmic pain is amenable to SCS while TCD pain cannot be effectively treated in this manner. Our findings imply that in patients in whom SCS is successful, the pathology is likely to be either spinal or peripheral, and the effectiveness of SCS derives from the locally-induced activation of inhibitory interneurons as described in the Gate-Control theory.[30] In contrast, in patients in whom SCS fails, our evidence shows that the pathology is thalamocortical, and the distant induction of dorsal column depolarization provided by SCS is insufficient to effectively modify thalamocortical physiology. The results underline the fundamental differences between peripheral and centrally generated nociception.

COMPLEX REGIONAL PAIN SYNDROME

MEG recordings were made in 11 patients with complex regional pain syndrome (CRPS) type I.[17] This disorder is a chronic progressive disease characterized by severe pain, swelling, and changes in the skin in the region of pain. The absence of a nerve lesion distinguish Type I from Type II.

MEG Power Spectra and Localization of Low Frequency Sources

As in the other MEG recordings of spontaneous activity in patients with neuropathic pain, the power spectra in these patients were characterized by the presence of activity in the theta range. Activity in the delta range was also remarked in seven of the 11 people in this group.[17]

Independent component analysis revealed that every patient had independent sources of theta band activity localized to somatosensory cortex. These localizations were in somatotopic agreement with pain localization. In addition, every patient had sources of activity in the delta (4–8 Hz) frequency range that were localized bilaterally to mesial orbito-frontal cortex and frontal pole.[17]

INTRAOPERATIVE RECORDINGS AND THALAMIC LESIONS

Jeanmonod and his group have carried out a series of studies that included intraoperative recordings of thalamic activity before and after central lateral thalamotomy (CLT) in patients with neuropathic pain.[14,15,31] Using single unit thalamic recordings they found that >99% of the cells did not respond to somatosensory or motor stimulation.[10,31] About half (45–50%) of these unresponsive cells were characterized by low frequency rhythmic firing consistent with the presence of low threshold calcium bursts. After CLT 67% of the patients reported complete (100%) or good (50–99%) pain relief with no somatosensory deficits.[10,31] The most effective pain relief was found in those patients with colocalization of bursting with the lesion site.[31]

Increased low frequency activity was also seen in pain patients at the level of the cortex. The dominant frequency of the EEG power spectra was shifted to lower frequencies in the patient group compared to controls.[14,15] The maximum difference between the two groups was seen at 6-9 Hz and was localized to prefrontal medial, cingulate, as well as somatosensory regions of the pain matrix.[15] EEG recordings made 12 months after the CLT showed a median pain relief of 95% with decreased low frequency activity in anterior cingulate.[14,15] Beta range activity was also increased in the patient group.[14,15] Frontal regions contributed most to this increase and coherence analysis found coupling between the theta and beta range frequencies in the patient group.[14] This is consistent with the "edge effect" aspect of thalamocortical dysthymia as given in the next section.

According to thalamocortical dysrhythmic hypothesis, a switch in the intrinsic firing pattern of thalamic cells from tonic to phasic and the establishment of a reciprocal thalamocortical loop underlies the increases in low frequency activity seen in MEG and EEG recordings from pain patients.[11,14,15,16,32] This was tested directly in a study combining local field potential (LFP) recordings from posterior central lateral thalamic nucleus (CL) with EEG in 10 neurogenic pain patients.[13] A theta peak was present in the LFP of all the patients and dominated the EEG spectrum in six patients. The coherence between the thalamus and cortex was strongest in the 4–9 Hz frequency range in all of the patients. Its magnitude was comparable to that between EEG electrode pairs separated by intermediate or long distances. The highest theta band coherence was between the CL and frontal EEG electrodes. This frontal localization overlaps with the region of increased theta activation seen in EEG[14,15,33] and MEG[16,17] recordings from pain patients and participate in the cortical pain matrix.[34–38]

Consistent with this view and with the correlation between low frequency activity and subjective pain experience is the fact that clinical improvement has been correlated with a reduction of low frequency cortical activity. For example, reduction of neuropathic pain sensation following transcranial magnetic stimulation is concomitant with a reduction of low frequency activity and pre-existing TCD electrical abnormalities have been attenuated after SCS leading to pain relief.[16] These results are similar to those found in tinnitus cases.[39,40] Moreover, such sound masking resulting in the disappearance of the tinnitus is accompanied by the mark reduction, or total abolition, of the low frequency signature within the auditory cortex.[27,41]

HIGH FREQUENCY FIRING AND THE EDGE EFFECT

On the cortical level, during normal high-frequency cortical activity, Layer III–IV cortical interneurons release GABA onto neighboring cells, in a process termed lateral inhibition.[42] It is hypothesized that under normal conditions, a given region of cortex activated in the gamma range inhibits other gamma activity from occurring in its periphery. However, in TCD, where projections from thalamus entrain a core of low-frequency cortical activity, lateral inhibition is abolished due to the lower rate of firing. Thus, in the region surrounding the core of theta activity, ectopic gamma activity can occur and cause pain to be perceived if this activity is in pain-related cortical areas.[11]

This "edge effect"[27] was first described in the retina by Hartline.[43] Harline found that when a given region of *limulus* retina is activated, a reduction of lateral inhibition creates a physiological border between activated and silent zones. There is a serious possibility that an analogous mechanism exists in the thalamocortical system creating regions underlying positive symptoms of pain and allodynia, in addition to being a possible underlying mechanism for negative symptoms seen in movements or psychiatric disorders.[44,45]

Such an effect has also been shown in tinnitus patients,[46,47] and in those with central pain,[13] and in an animal model.[45] Recent MEG recordings from patients with trigeminal neuralgia pain have demonstrated co-localization of theta (Figure 4.3A) and gamma band (Figure 4.3B) activity.[48] Animal experiments using voltage-sensitive dye in deafferented cortex supports the concept that disconnection-induced hyperpolarization of thalamocortical modules leads to the deinactivation of T-type Ca^{++} channels and low-threshold spike activity, accompanied by adjacent increases in high-frequency firing.[49]

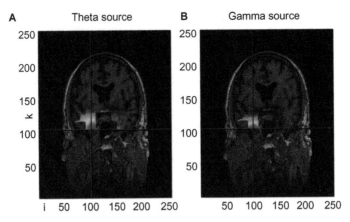

FIGURE 4.3   Example of localization of theta and gamma activity in a patient with trigeminal neuralgia pain. Localization of a source theta band **A** (4–8 Hz) and gamma band **B** activity (35–55 Hz) in orbital frontal region on patient's MRI. Such co-localization is consistent with high frequency activity adjacent to low frequency activity according to the edge effect in thalamocortical dysrhythmia.

DISCUSSION

The findings summarized here extend the original conception of Head and Holmes,[50] who first suggested the relevance of an "essential thalamic structure" (i.e., a central generator) for neuropathic pain. In addition to this early model, ample recent evidence exists for changes in thalamic physiology in subjects with neuropathic pain. As summarized above, several investigators have noted bursting activity in medial and lateral thalami of awake chronic pain patients during surgical recordings.[10,12,31,51,52] Disturbance in thalamocortical interplay has been consistently found in other neuropathic central pain states such as following spinal cord injury,[53] chronic low back pain,[54] and even in chronic visceral pain conditions.[55] In addition, EEG and thalamic activity have a high temporal coherence in the theta band in these patients.[13,14] Thus, there is an emerging theme of TCD in neuropathic pain states.

These data correlate well with findings obtained with functional MRI, PET and SPECT.[37,56,57] A positron emission tomography (PET) study by Iadarola and colleagues[58] identified a consistent decrease in thalamic metabolism contralateral to painful limbs in subjects whose pain was presumed to have a central source. Recent studies have reported metabolic differences in thalamus[59] and in anterior cingulate cortex[60] between spinal cord injury patients with chronic neuropathic pain and pain-free healthy controls. While the precise correlation between oscillatory frequency and hemodynamics remains an area of active study, it has been suggested that a decrease in thalamic oscillatory frequency—here, from the gamma (30–50 Hz) to the theta (4–8 Hz) range—could be reflected by locally diminished perfusion.[61] Analogously, a correlation between neuronal firing rates within the internal segment of the globus pallidus and thalamic positive emission tomography (PET) activity in patients suffering from Parkinson's disease—another manifestation of thalamocortical dysrhythmia—has been well described.[62]

Pain Treatment and Thalamocortical Dysrhythmia

Successful treatment has also been accomplished in other instances of TCD—particularly in Parkinson's disease—through the implantation of deep-brain stimulators.[63] The effectiveness of this therapy is consistent with the mechanisms postulated: high-frequency stimulation could raise the resting potential of RT or intralaminar neurons above the level of T-type Ca^{++} channel deinactivation. Alternatively, deep-brain stimulation may inhibit its target by one of several possible mechanisms. In this scenario, as the physiological hyperpolarizing output of the basal ganglia is inhibited, the thalamus is released from hyperinhibition and low threshold spikes are abolished as thalamic neuron resting potentials return to the normal waking range.

The effectiveness of motor cortex stimulation in treating some cases of neuropathic pain[64,65,66,67] may also be understood as resulting from top-down thalamic depolarization. It should be noted that the qualified success of this approach speaks to the challenge of modifying the thalamocortical loop using a depolarizer effectively situated outside the system. In our recordings, the subject with both sensory and limbic sources failed a technically successful trial of motor cortex stimulation, an outcome that further emphasizes the difficulty of modulating widespread dysrhythmia from a single cortical location. It should also be noted that the established technique of electroconvulsive therapy and more recent advances using transcranial magnetic stimulation[65] might similarly derive their effectiveness from a temporary rise in the resting potential of thalamic cells.

In addition to these successes, some of the therapeutic failures for chronic pain also lend support to the theory that deafferentation pain can be related to a centrally generated hyperpolarization. For example, the finding that sensory blockade is known to increase pain in some patients,[68] coupled with the low success rate for surgical tractotomy,[69] are consistent with a paradigm in which the additional sensory blockade actually deafferents the thalamus even further and adds to the disfacilitation which causes LTS bursts. Conversely, some patients with plexus avulsions report pain reduction with sensory input to the affected limb. This presumably activates the thalamus, temporarily counteracting the deafferentation effects. These findings, together with the reported effectiveness of transcutaneous electrical neurostimulation (TENS) in some cases,[70,71] is supported by a model in which increased input to the thalamus restores a more depolarized CNS mode.

It should be noted that TCD is one of a variety of mechanisms that can underlie central pain. And the question of which acute pain events will ultimately become neuropathic pain of some form remains a topic of investigation. In the realm of dysrhythmic pain (and other thalamocortical dysrhythmias) these factors remain to be elucidated, though it is possible to speculate on several potential factors which could, either alone or in combination, lead to persistently aberrant activity. Perhaps the most obvious potential locus of pathology is the T-type Ca^{++} channel itself. In some individuals and/or situations, channel isoforms that are more readily deinactivated (and therefore predispose the system to low threshold spikes) may be expressed. A wide range of other ionic mechanisms, for example, specific hyperpolarizing combinations of K^+ leakage channels, could also be involved. In addition, issues related to individual anatomical connectivity might be significant in TCD pain states, such that congenital neuronal or synaptic sparseness could predispose an individual to deafferentation-mediated hyperpolarization.

A fundamental issue to be considered here is that of sensory binding and its functional correlates. This essay presents a set of electrophysiological findings that indicate that pain, in this case central pain, is correlated with two distinct electrophysiological components, one that defines the localization on the body of the pain experience and, as such, is *sui generis* for each patient and one that is similar and omnipresent in all patients. While the former signature is indeed a description of location the latter relates to the emotional sensation of pain, as it is common to all patients and is reduced by procedures that obliterate the emotional component of the sensation, that is the hurt. It is very clear that the unpleasant sensation/emotion of being hurt happens without actual localization as, for instance, with moral pain or as it happens with other emotions, for instance fear. Having fear localized to ones hand would be of no survival value while localizing 'nociceptive' pain is invaluable for survival. As such then a careful analysis of issues as temporal coherence between low frequencies in localized pain *versus* non coherent activity between simultaneous but unrelated stimuli may go a long way in clarifying he electrophysiological mechanism for temporal binding.

References

1. Connors BW, Gutnick MJ. Intrinsic firing patterns of diverse neocortical neurons [see comment]. *Trends Neurosci.* 1990;13:99–104.
2. Getting PA. Emerging principles governing the operation of neural networks. *Annu Rev Neurosci.* 1989;12:185–204.

3. Llinas RR. The intrinsic electrophysiological properties of mammalian neurons: insights into central nervous system function. *Science.* 1988;242:1654–1664.
4. Margolis DJ, Detwiler PB. Different mechanisms generate maintained activity in ON and OFF retinal ganglion cells. *J Neurosci.* 2007;27:5994–6005.
5. Turrigiano G, Abbott LF, Marder E. Activity-dependent changes in the intrinsic properties of cultured neurons. *Science.* 1994;264:974–977.
6. Llinas R, Greenfield SA, Jahnsen H. Electrophysiology of pars compacta cells in the in vitro substantia nigra–a possible mechanism for dendritic release. *Brain Res.* 1984;294:127–132.
7. Llinas R, Jahnsen H. Electrophysiology of mammalian thalamic neurones in vitro. *Nature.* 1982;297:406–408.
8. Jones E. *The Thalamus.* New York: Cambridge University Press; 2007.
9. Steriade M, Llinas RR. The functional states of the thalamus and the associated neuronal interplay. *Physiol Rev.* 1988;68:649–742.
10. Jeanmonod D, Magnin M, Morel A. Low-threshold calcium spike bursts in the human thalamus. Common physiopathology for sensory, motor and limbic positive symptoms. *Brain.* 1996;119:363–375.
11. Llinas RR, Ribary U, Jeanmonod D, Kronberg E, Mitra PP. Thalamocortical dysrhythmia: a neurological and neuropsychiatric syndrome characterized by magnetoencephalography. *Proc Natl Acad Sci U S A.* 1999;96:15222–15227.
12. Lenz FA, Kwan HC, Dostrovsky JO, Tasker RR. Characteristics of the bursting pattern of action potentials that occurs in the thalamus of patients with central pain. *Brain Res.* 1989;496:357–360.
13. Sarnthein J, Jeanmonod D. High thalamocortical theta coherence in patients with neurogenic pain. *Neuroimage.* 2008;39:1910–1917.
14. Sarnthein J, Stern J, Aufenberg C, Rousson V, Jeanmonod D. Increased EEG power and slowed dominant frequency in patients with neurogenic pain. *Brain.* 2006;129:55–64.
15. Stern J, Jeanmonod D, Sarnthein J. Persistent EEG overactivation in the cortical pain matrix of neurogenic pain patients. *Neuroimage.* 2006;31:721–731.
16. Schulman JJ, Zonenshayn M, Ramirez RR, Ribary U, Llinas R. Thalamocortical dysrhythmia syndrome: MEG imaging of neuropathic pain. *Thal Rel Sys.* 2005;3:33–39.
17. Walton KD, Dubois M, Llinas RR. Abnormal thalamocortical activity in patients with Complex Regional Pain Syndrome (CRPS) type I. *Pain.* 2010;150:41–51.
18. Wydenkeller S, Maurizio S, Dietz V, Halder P. Neuropathic pain in spinal cord injury: significance of clinical and electrophysiological measures. *Eur J Neurosci.* 2009;30:91–99.
19. Inui K, Tsuji T, Kakigi R. Temporal analysis of cortical mechanisms for pain relief by tactile stimuli in humans. *Cerebral Cortex.* 2006;16:355–365.
20. Somers DL, Somers MF. Treatment of neuropathic pain in a patient with diabetic neuropathy using transcutaneous electrical nerve stimulation applied to the skin of the lumbar region. *Phys Ther.* 1999;79:767–775.
21. Llinás RR, Ribary U, Joliot M, Wang Y. Content and context in temporal thalamocortical binding. In: Buzsaki G, Llinás RR, Singer W, Berthoz A, Christen Y, eds. *Temporal Coding in the Brain.* Berlin, Heidelberg: Springer-Verlag; 1994. p. 251–272.
22. Gerke MB, Duggan AW, Xu L, Siddall PJ. Thalamic neuronal activity in rats with mechanical allodynia following contusive spinal cord injury. *Neurosci.* 2003;117:715–722.
23. Kim J, Jung JI, Na HS, Hong SK, Yoon YW. Effects of morphine on mechanical allodynia in a rat model of central neuropathic pain. *Neuroreport.* 2003;14:1017–1020.
24. Wang G, Thompson SM. Maladaptive homeostatic plasticity in a rodent model of central pain syndrome: thalamic hyperexcitability after spinothalamic tract lesions. *J Neurosci.* 2008;28:11959–11969.

25. Marini G, Ceccarelli P, Mancia M. Thalamocortical dysrhythmia and the thalamic reticular nucleus in behaving rats. *Clin Neurophysiol.* 2002;113:1152–1164.
26. Dejerine J, Roussy G. Le syndome thalamique. *Rev Neurol (Paris).* 1906;14:521–532.
27. Llinas R, Urbano F, Leznik E, Ramizeriz R, Van Marle H. Rhythmic and dysrhythmic thalamocortical dynamics: GABA systems and the edge effect. *Trends Neurosci.* 2005;28:325–333.
28. Grachev ID, Fredrickson BE, Apkarian AV. Brain chemistry reflects dual states of pain and anxiety in chronic low back pain. *J Neural Transm.* 2002;109:1309–1334.
29. Penfield W. The excitable cortex in conscious man *The Sherrington Lectures*, 5. Springfield, Ill: C.C. Thomas; 1958. pp. 17.
30. Melzack R, Wall PD. Pain mechanisms: a new theory. *Science.* 1965;150:971–979.
31. Jeanmonod D, Magnin M, Morel A. Thalamus and neurogenic pain: physiological, anatomical and clinical data. [erratum appears in Neuroreport 1993 Aug;4(8):1066]. *Neuroreport.* 1993;4:475–478.
32. Gucer G, Niedermeyer E, Long DM. Thalamic EEG recordings in patients with chronic pain. *J Neurol.* 1978;219:47–61.
33. Prichep LS, John ER, Howard B, Merkin H, Hiesiger EM. Evaluation of the pain matrix using EEG source localization: a feasibility study. *Pain med.* 2011;12:1241–1248.
34. Apkarian AV, Bushnell MC, Treede RD, Zubieta JK. Human brain mechanisms of pain perception and regulation in health and disease. *Eur J Pain.* 2005;9:463–484.
35. Duerden EG, Albanese MC. Localization of pain-related brain activation: a meta-analysis of neuroimaging data. *Hum Brain Mapp.* 2011.
36. Jones AK, Kulkarni B, Derbyshire SW. Pain mechanisms and their disorders: imaging in clinical neuroscience. *Br Med Bull.* 2003;65:83–93.
37. Peyron R, Laurent B, Garcia-Larrea L. Functional imaging of brain responses to pain. A review and meta-analysis (2000). *Neurophysiol Clin.* 2000;30:263–288.
38. Treede RD, Kenshalo DR, Gracely RH, Jones AK. The cortical representation of pain. *Pain.* 1999;79:105–111.
39. De Ridder D, De Mulder G, Verstraeten E, et al. Auditory cortex stimulation for tinnitus. *Acta Neurochir Suppl.* 2007;97:451–462.
40. Richter GT, Mennemeier M, Bartel T, et al. Repetitive transcranial magnetic stimulation for tinnitus: a case study. *Laryngoscope.* 2006;116:1867–1872.
41. Tyler R. *Tinnitus Handbook.* San Diego: Singular Publishing Group; 2000.
42. Beierlein M, Gibson JR, Connors BW. A network of electrically coupled interneurons drives synchronized inhibition in neocortex. *Nat Neurosci.* 2000;3:904–910.
43. Hartline HK. Visual receptors and retinal interaction *Nobel Lectures.* Amsterdam: Elsevier; 1967.
44. Llinas R, Ribary U, Jeanmonod D, et al. Thalamocortical dysrhythmia I. Functional and imaging aspects. *Thal Rel Sys.* 2001;1:237–244.
45. Llinas RR, Choi S, Urbano FJ, Shin HS. Gamma-band deficiency and abnormal thalamocortical activity in P/Q-type channel mutant mice [see comment]. *Proc Natl Acad Sci U S A.* 2007;104:17819–17824.
46. De Ridder D, van der Loo E, Van der Kelen K, Menovsky T, van de Heyning P, Moller A. Theta, alpha and beta burst transcranial magnetic stimulation: brain modulation in tinnitus. *Int J Med Sci.* 2007;4:237–241.
47. Weisz N, Moratti S, Meinzer M, Dohrmann K, Elbert T. Tinnitus perception and distress is related to abnormal spontaneous brain activity as measured by magnetoencephalography. *PLoS Med.* 2005;2:e153.
48. Walton K, Garcia JR, Rabello G, Delfino J, Llinas R. 2012. Theta and gamma oscillations typical of thalamocortical dysrhythmia in patients with trigeminal neuralgia pain In Neuroscience Meeting Planner, Program No 31802. Society for Neuroscience, New Orleans, LA.

49. Leznik E, Makarenko V, Llinas R. Electrotonically mediated oscillatory patterns in neuronal ensembles: an in vitro voltage-dependent dye-imaging study in the inferior olive. *J Neurosci*. 2002;22:2804–2815.

50. Head H, Holmes G. Sensory disturbances from cerebral lesions. *Brain*. 1911;34:102–254.

51. Hirayama T, Dostrovsky JO, Gorecki J, Tasker RR, Lenz FA. Recordings of abnormal activity in patients with deafferentation and central pain. *Stereotact Funct Neurosurg*. 1989;52:120–126.

52. Rinaldi PC, Young RF, Albe-Fessard D, Chodakiewitz J. Spontaneous neuronal hyperactivity in the medial and intralaminar thalamic nuclei of patients with deafferentation pain. *J Neurosurg*. 1991;74:415–421.

53. Boord P, Siddall PJ, Tran Y, Herbert D, Middleton J, Craig A. Electroencephalographic slowing and reduced reactivity in neuropathic pain following spinal cord injury. *Spinal Cord*. 2008;46:118–123.

54. Baliki MN, Chialvo DR, Geha PY, et al. Chronic pain and the emotional brain: specific brain activity associated with spontaneous fluctuations of intensity of chronic back pain. *J Neurosci*. 2006;26:12165–12173.

55. Drewes A, Gratkowski M, Sami S, Dimcevski G, Funch-Jensen P, Arendt-Nielsen L. Is the pain in chronic pancreatitis of neuropathic origin? support from EEG studies during experimental pain. *World J Gastroenterol*. 2008;14:4020–4027.

56. Moisset X, Bouhassira D. Brain imaging of neuropathic pain. *Neuroimage*. 2007;37(Suppl 1):S80–S88.

57. Wu CT, Fan YM, Sun CM, et al. Correlation between changes in regional cerebral blood flow and pain relief in complex regional pain syndrome type 1. *Clin Nucl Med*. 2006;31:317–320.

58. Iadarola MJ, Max MB, Berman KF, et al. Unilateral decrease in thalamic activity observed with positron emission tomography in patients with chronic neuropathic pain. *Pain*. 1995;63:55–64.

59. Pattany PM, Yezierski RP, Widerstrom-Noga EG, et al. Proton magnetic resonance spectroscopy of the thalamus in patients with chronic neuropathic pain after spinal cord injury. *AJNR Am J Neuroradiol*. 2002;23:901–905.

60. Widerstrom-Noga E, Pattany PM, Cruz-Almeida Y, et al. Metabolite concentrations in the anterior cingulate cortex predict high neuropathic pain impact after spinal cord injury. *Pain*. 2012

61. Schiff ND, Ribary U, Moreno DR, et al. Residual cerebral activity and behavioural fragments can remain in the persistently vegetative brain. *Brain*. 2002;125:1210–1234.

62. Eidelberg D, Moeller JR, Kazumata K, et al. Metabolic correlates of pallidal neuronal activity in Parkinson's disease. *Brain*. 1997;120:1315–1324. Pt 8.

63. Benabid AL, Vercucil L, Benazzouz A, et al. Deep brain stimulation: what does it offer?. *Adv Neurol*. 2003;91:293–302.

64. Delavallee M, Abu-Serieh B, de Tourchaninoff M, Raftopoulos C. Subdural motor cortex stimulation for central and peripheral neuropathic pain: a long-term follow-up study in a series of eight patients. *Neurosurgery*. 2008;63:101–105. [discussion 105–108].

65. Hosomi K, Saitoh Y, Kishima H, et al. Electrical stimulation of primary motor cortex within the central sulcus for intractable neuropathic pain. *Clin Neurophysiol*. 2008;119:993–1001.

66. Stadler 3rd JA, Ellens DJ, Rosenow JM. Deep brain stimulation and motor cortical stimulation for neuropathic pain. *Curr Pain Headache Rep*. 2011;15:8–13.

67. Tanei T, Kajita Y, Noda H, et al. Efficacy of motor cortex stimulation for intractable central neuropathic pain: comparison of stimulation parameters between post-stroke pain and other central pain. *Neurol Med Chir (Tokyo)*. 2011;51:8–14.

68. Bonica J. Pain management: past and current status. In: Stanley T, Fine P, eds. *Anesthesiology and Pain Management*. Boston: Kluwer Academic; 1991.

69. Tasker R. Surgical approaches to chronic pain. In: Portenoy R, ed. *Pain Management: Theory and Practice.* Philadelphia: F.A. Davis; 1996. p. 290–311.
70. Loeser JM. Transcutaneous electrical stimulation for pain relief. *Acta Anaesthesiol Belg.* 1984;35:243–248.
71. Sjolund B. Role of transcutaneous electrical nerve stimulation, central nervous system stimulation, and ablative procedures in central pain syndromes. In: Casey K, ed. *Pain and Central Nervous System Disease: The Central Pain Syndromes.* New York: Raven Press; 1991. p. 267–274.

5

Surgical Interventions for Pain

Daniel M. Aghion and Garth Rees Cosgrove

Department of Neurosurgery Rhode Island Hospital and Hasbro Children's
Hospital and Brown University, Alpert School of Medicine, Providence,
RI, USA

To understand the surgical interventions possible to alleviate or even eliminate pain, a basic understanding of the physiology and anatomy of nociception must be appreciated.

All tissues of the body are innervated by nociceptors with the exception of the neuraxis. These are primary afferent neurons that are specialized to detect the presence, intensity and quality of noxious stimuli. The somas or cell bodies of these primary afferent neurons are located in the dorsal root ganglia and trigeminal ganglia, and their innervations follow segmental dermatomes. The vast majority of nociceptive sensory endings are supplied by small diameter axons, which are either very thinly myelinated or not myelinated at all. These dorsal root ganglia axons aggregate in the lateral aspect of the dorsal root, and then, upon entry into the spinal cord either send a primary projection directly into the dorsal horn at the segment of entry, or they form branches that project over 1–2 segments through Lissauer's tract and the dorsal columns. After initial synaptic processing, the nociceptive information is carried to the brain by direct axonal projections to the thalamus, brainstem, hypothalamus, and forebrain. This is done via the spinothalamic tract, spinoreticular tract, and spinohypothalamic tract respectively. Incoming nociceptive information is processed centrally by several cortical structures including primary somatosensory cortex, secondary somatosensory cortex, anterior cingulate cortex, and insular cortex.

Primary sensory cortex mainly receives direct nociceptive input from the ipsilateral ventral posterolateral (VPL) and ventral posteromedial (VPM) thalamus. Secondary somatosensory cortex receives input from the thalamic nuclei (VPL and VPM) or the medial ascending systems from the contralateral thalamus and is involved in spatially directed attention towards pain. The anterior cingulate cortex, part of the limbic system, receives input from the medial thalamic nuclei and is involved in the affective or emotional aspects of pain. The insular cortex, also having connections to the limbic system, receives nociceptive input via the medial spinothalamic system and is considered a multisensory area that integrates nociceptive, tactile, vestibular, and visceral sensations. Whether the character of one's pain is peripheral or central in nature, surgical interventions for pain may be performed at the level of the primary afferent neurons, through their ascending pathways, within the thalamus or in areas of the cortex that these fibers project to.

Unlike other physiological processes, pain does not emanate from a single specific organ but is a distributed system. There is also no completely objective way to know that pain truly exists nor a single target or location to treat it. Therefore, patient selection and psychological assessment is of the utmost importance in evaluating a patient for a surgical pain-relief procedure. An individual's integration and neural affective information is crucial to understanding their pain. Today, multidisciplinary pain centers treat all aspects of pain and include behavioral, cognitive, and affective components of their pain. Assessing each component of the pain is crucial when considering invasive options of treatment. Psychological testing is also warranted prior to proceeding with specific pain procedures because many patients may exhibit neurobehavioral deficits, depression, anxiety, somatoform disorders, factitious or malingering disorders, personality disorders, or even substance abuse. All of these co-morbidities should be treated before considering any surgical intervention.

NEUROSURGICAL PROCEDURES

When evaluating a patient with chronic pain and entertaining a surgical option, one practical approach to discriminate the types of procedures available is to divide them in to "Neuromodulation" and "Neuroablation" procedures. Neuroablation is typically a destructive procedure that interrupts afferent input from the nociceptive pathways or selectively ablates the thalamic and cortical areas that mediate perception of painful stimuli. Although the lesions themselves are irreversible, the long term effect on pain perception is often limited to months or years because of the adaptablitiy and plasticity of the nervous system. Neuromodulation on the other hand, seeks to decrease pain by modulating nociceptive input by either pharmacological or electrical means. This typically requires implantable pumps or electrical stimulating devices and has the advantage of testability, adjustability and reversibility. They tend to be very expensive in terms of equipment and medical follow-up.

Neuroablative procedures are generally simple, one-time procedures and tend to be much less costly. As mentioned previously, surgical interventions for pain may be performed at the level of the primary afferent neurons, through their ascending pathways, or in areas of the cortex that these fibers project to. In general, however, any surgical intervention must target at least one synaptic junction in the neuraxis proximal to the level of the injury or source of the pain. For example, for pain originating in a spinal nerve root or more peripherally, surgery must be directed to the spinal cord. Similarly, if the pain is the result of a spinal cord injury, interventions must focus on the thalamus or cortex. This is especially true for neuromodulation techniques.

NEUROMODULATION- RELIEVING PAIN BY MODULATING PAIN PATHWAYS

Peripheral Nerve Stimulation (PNS)

Limited publications are available on PNS, but it has been performed for over 30 years. Electric stimulation of peripheral nerves has been used for treatment of chronic pain arising from peripheral nerve trauma or entrapment with or without a sympathetic component. Electrodes are implanted proximal to the injury site and include ulnar, median, radial, and common peroneal nerves. Patient selection should include instances where pain arising from an identifiable nerve with temporary pain relief after selective nerve blocking techniques. The procedure is performed by exposing the desired section of peripheral nerve proximal to the injury, dissecting it completely from its surrounding tissue, placing the electrode lead under the exposed nerve so that all leads are in contact with the nerve, and securing it in place. The receiver is then placed in the anterior abdominal or chest wall. For lower extremity PNS, receivers are placed in the buttocks or lateral thigh. Voltage requirements range from 0.5 V to 3.0 V with pulse widths ranging from 120–400 microseconds and rates from 50–80 Hz. Either cycling or continuous stimulation modes are generally available for PNS. How PNS works to alleviate pain is unknown but it may be similar to SCS by modulating the painful afferent input and its processing and perception within the central nervous system.

Spinal Cord Stimulation (SCS)

SCS involves electrical stimulation of the posterior aspect of the spinal cord for the treatment of certain chronic pain conditions such as chronic neuropathic pain or failed back surgery syndrome. Some authors report the use of SCS for severe angina pectoris, ischemic pain, due to occlusive or vasospastic arterial disease, or phantom limb and stump pain. The neurophysiologic mechanisms of pain suppression by SCS are poorly understood but it should be applied with low intensity allowing activation of low-threshold, large-diameter fibers in the dorsal columns. In order for SCS to be successful, stimulation evoked paresthesias must be experienced in the entire painful area. Effective pain relief with SCS is most likely to occur in cases with neurogenic pain which is ongoing and spontaneous. Percutaneous catheter leads as well as paddle leads are available for trial or permanent implantation. The percutaneous approach is attractive because it allows for electrode insertion without muscle destruction or bony removal. Paddle electrodes require placement via a small laminotomy under direct visualization and can be passed in a cephalad or caudal direction. Paddle electrodes also have an insulated dorsal surface and usually tend to migrate less. The procedure is performed on an awake and cooperative patient to yield the best results. The receiver is placed in the infraclavicular area, abdominal or chest wall, or buttock region. Stimulation can be given in increments of 0.1 V and with rates up to 130 Hz. Radiofrequency coupled systems can deliver stimulation with a rate up to 1400 Hz and the patient may have full access to the parameters of stimulation.

Deep Brain Stimulation (DBS)

Currently, the most common application of DBS is for Parkinson's disease, where the globus pallidus or subthalamic nucleus is stimulated. Chronic stimulation of subcortical brain structures is becoming an increasingly popular mode of therapy in functional neurosurgery. Though the exact mechanism of DBS is unknown, theories implicate a depolarizing blockade of neurons when stimulated at high frequencies. This is supported by high frequency stimulation (>100 Hz) producing a similar effect to lesioning that structure. Whereas high frequency stimulation is routinely used in movement disorder DBS, lower frequency stimulation has been shown to be efficacious in pain surgery. In the early 1950s electrodes placed in the septum pellucidum were used to treat schizophrenia and metastatic carcinomas and provided good pain relief. Pain relief lasted for up to eight hours even after the stimulator was turned off. In today's age, modern day DBS targets for pain syndromes are the periventricular gray (PVG), periaqueductal gray (PAG), or thalamic, medial lemniscus, and internal capsule. Targets in the thalamus are the VPM for chronic intractable facial pain, or VPL for similar chronic deafferentation pain in the extremities. Similarly, the posterior limb of the internal capsule has been stimulated using DBS methods and has been shown to provide good pain relief. Mixed pain syndrome patients should undergo implantation of both PVG and thalamic electrodes. Around the same time that these experiments were being pursued, it was noted that the lateral margin of the PAG could be stimulated in animals, allowing for awake, intra-abdominal surgery to be performed. This was then confirmed in humans where 10–75 Hz DBS was delivered to the PAG and PVG regions providing with good pain relief. Some pain conditions treated with DBS are thalamic syndromes, brachial plexus avulsions, postcordotomy dysesthesias, spinal cord injuries, and cancer pain.

Prior to offering DBS to treat chronic pain, appropriate selection criteria must be applied and psychiatric evaluation is mandatory. DBS for chronic pain should be used only in patients who are incapacitated and have failed to respond to all other treatment modalities. Pain must be the predominant complaint and they must understand that the procedure is not curative. The goal with DBS for chronic pain is a 50% reduction in pain. Additionally, patients must understand that pain recurrence is common.

Patients undergo application of a stereotactic head frame followed by CT or MRI, and anatomic target localization is performed using standardized anatomic brain atlases with relation to the anterior commisure and posterior commisure. Under local anaesthesia, a burr hole is made 2.5 cm lateral to the midline and using stereotactic coordinates, the anatomical targets are chosen. A blunt-tipped stylet is then introduced stereotactically into the brain parenchyma 10 mm proximal to the chosen target and physiological localization by way of recording is performed. Physiologic localization is helpful for definitive target determination in most targets for pain because of the frequent discrepancy between the expected location and actual position of the targets. Optimal location for the DBS electrode(s) is determined and the lead is then secured in place (Figure 5.1). Patients undergo a trial period for three to seven days where various stimulation parameters are used and a detailed pain diary is kept by the patient. Typical stimulation parameters include unipolar or bipolar stimulation with 25–75 Hz and pulse widths of 60–500 microsec. A successful trial period consists of >50% reduction in pain with stimulation. Pulse generator implantation is usually carried out at a secondary surgery under general anesthesia where the receiver is implanted in the infraclavicular region.

Motor Cortex Stimulation (MCS)

According to Takashi Tsubokawa, the term central deafferentation pain is used to refer to pain in which the flow of afferent nerve impulses has been partially or completely interrupted at the neospinothalamic system within the CNS. This too is a neurogenic pain that involves a lesion distal to the dorsal column pathway, such as in the thalamocortical tracts,

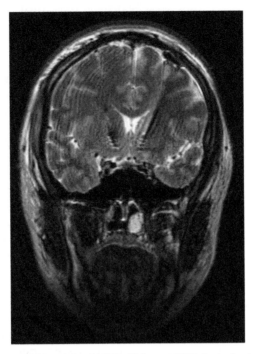

FIGURE 5.1   Coronal T1 weighted MRI of bilateral DBS electrodes in the ventral striatum of a patient with intractable atypical facial pain.

and is treated by MCS. Classically, this type of pain is resistant to morphine treatment but not to barbiturates. The typical population is stroke
patients where there is absence of sensory input into the somatosensory cortex producing hyperactivity in the neurons of the afferent pain
pathway above the level of the lesion. Surgery modulating these areas,
by way of MCS, has been shown to provide relief in this type of deafferentation pain. The procedure involves identifying the motor cortex
on the superficial skull then performing a craniotomy exposing the dura
overlying the motor cortex involved in the painful area and placing the
electrodes adjacent to this. At this point, low frequency stimulation is
provided and muscle contraction in the target region is observed. The
delivered stimuli are monophasic with a duration of 0.1–0.5 msec and
applied continuously for 10–20 minutes. As with other pain procedures,
test stimulation is also performed with MCS and no stimulation is given
at night. Care must be taken to perform low frequency stimulation as the
motor cortex is susceptible to habituation, and high frequency cortical
stimulation can cause seizures. The effect on sensory function that MCS
has is a sensation of light tingling or vibration in the same area where the
patients reported pain. This stimulation occurred at an intensity below

the threshold for muscle contraction. If adequate relief is provided, then through secondary surgery, the stimulator is internalized after one week of testing and patients can select varying stimulation parameter frequencies, 5–12 Hz over 0.5 msec. Interestingly, some patients with thalamic pain caused by hemorrhage or stroke have reported unexpected improvement in their motor deficits. This appears to be related to an inhibition of their rigidity and can even be seen in some Parkinson's patients that have undergone MCS. In summary, MCS can control central deafferentation pain in ~50% of treated patients that do not suffer from severe motor disturbances (also see Chapter 7 by Masri and Keller in this book).

Intrathecal Opioids

Intrathecal (IT) administration of opioids is the classic example of a neuroaugmentive procedure. Where electrical stimulation is not indicated or complications of neuroablative procedures are significant, chronic, intrathecal infusion of analgesics are often effective in controlling intractable pain. The analgesic effect of IT opioids is achieved through spinal and supraspinal opioid receptors with minimal influence on motor, sensory, and sympathetic reflexes. IT morphine is the drug of choice and produces fewer adverse effects than its systemic administration in equianalgesic doses. Patient selection criteria for IT opioids are critical and careful diagnostic evaluations of the patient must be performed. Indications for IT opioid administration include known physiological source of pain, failure of maximal medical therapy, favorable psychosocial evaluation, and good response to IT opioid trial. Contraindications to this procedure are infection, uncorrectable coagulopathy, allergy to opioid agent going to be used, CSF obstruction, and severely limited life expectancy. Some reports also suggest that somatic pain was much more likely to be successfully treated by IT opioid administration than visceral pain. Several types of delivery systems are available for IT opioid administration and include short term intraspinal catheters, tunneled IT catheters, and fully implantable systems. All types of systems require an IT catheter which is made of silicone and is implanted through direct spinal puncture into the subarachnoid space. The catheter is advanced to the determined location and anchored to the dorsal fascia. This catheter is then tunneled to the subcutaneous anterior abdominal wall where it is connected to the programmable pump. This pump serves as the medication reservoir and is accessible percutaneously for medication refilling in a clinic, office, or even residential setting. Electronic interrogation and programming of the pump takes place percutaneously as well and the mode of infusion and dose may be altered at this time. With good patient selection criteria, success rates for

IT opioid administration are to the order of 70–80% with cancer patients, and 65–75% with nonmalignant chronic neuropathic pain.

NEUROABLATION- RELIEVING PAIN BY INTERRUPTING PAIN PATHWAYS

Neurectomy

A neurectomy is the transection or partial resection of a nerve. This can only be considered for small peripheral nerves that are purely sensory. This imparts complete numbness in the distributon of the nerve but can be useful in the face especially in trigger point areas. Unfortunately, it rarely provides long-lasting relief. Partial resection of a nerve is generally only considered for painful neuromas. The correct nerve is identified, the end-bulb neuroma is resected, and the proximal nerve is relocated to a site that is away from any irritation, usually into a nearby muscle.

Facet Blocks and Denervations

Low back pain and lumbar spondylosis is a disease that plagues a significant amount of the population. For years, the lumbar zygopophyseal joints have been targeted as both a diagnostic and therapeutic site for anesthetic injections for the pain they are associated with. Disc space narrowing occurs as the disc degenerates and becomes dehydrated. This leads to abnormal motion which produces osteophyte formation and inflammation within the facet joints and a gradual worsening of symptoms. For thoraco-lumbar injections, the patient is positioned prone and fluoroscopic imaging used to view the targeted joint. After the skin is anesthetized, a 22-guage, 3.5 inch spinal needle is advanced to the joint. 1.0–1.5 cc of local anesthetic with or without steroids is delivered. Volumes larger than this can rupture the facet capsule and spill over into the epidural space. Complications from facet blocks are infrequent and transient. Increase in pain and inadvertent intrathecal injection have been reported in the thoraco-lumbar spine, while vertebral artery puncture and strokes have been reported in the cervical region. Facet blocks can have both diagnostic and short term therapeutic value lasting a few weeks to months but often need to be repeated. If the facet block provides significant local back pain relief then a more enduring albeit not permanent relief can be achieved with facet rhizotomy. This procedure is performed by either radiofrequency ablation or cryoneurolysis and involves destruction of the medial and lateral nerve branches that innervate the facet.

Dorsal Root Ganglionectomy (DRG), Dorsal Rhizotomy (DR) and Dorsal Root Entry Zone (DREZ) Lesions

The nerve cell bodies of the nociceptive neurons reside in the dorsal root ganglion. Three to ten posterior spinal rootlets enter the posterolateral sulcus of the spinal cord creating what is thought of classically as the dorsal root entry zone (DREZ). This zone subserves pain perception for that dermatomal distrubtion but most areas of the body and peripheral nerves are innervated by multiple overlapping nerve roots. For this reason, both procedures also usually require lesioning at multiple levels for adequate pain relief. DRG and DR are sometimes indicated in patients suffering from chronic pain in a particular dermatomal distribution related to cancer or tumor.

DRG is still utilized in the cervical region for severe and intractable occipital neuralgia, where the C2 ganglion is removed with good long term results. Dorsal Rhizotomy is most often performed intradurally but may also be carried out extradurally. Intradural technique is performed through standard multi-level laminectomies allowing for overlap of innervations, and after the dura is opened, the selected sensory roots are followed rostrally to their respective true level and then cauterized, and transected. This technique however causes a loss of all sensation within that dermatome. Therefore, modifications of the DR were developed to preserve cutaneous and proprioceptive sensation namely the selective DR and the DREZ lesion.

Selective DR involves making small 1–2 mm incisions in to the ventral aspect of the DREZ thereby interrupting small unmyelinated nociceptive fibres while preserving larger heavily myelinated fibres subserving touch and proprioception which enter the DREZ dorsally. It does require a multilevel laminectomy and after the dura is opened, the arachnoid layers must be freed exposing rootlets and the pia mater. The microsurgical dissection then involves creating a longitudinal incision of the dorsolateral sulcus, ventrolaterally to the entry of the rootlets into the sulcus. Microbipolar cautery can then be performed within the sulcus down to the apex of the dorsal horn in the spinal segments targeted. The average lesion is 2–3 mm deep and at a 35 degree angle medially and ventrally. Lesions are performed at each selected level that corresponds to the pain dermatome.

DREZ lesions can also be performed using a small radiofrequency needle placed 2–3 mm into the DREZ area of the spinal cord through its dorsal surface. The tip is heated to 65–70 degrees centigrade thereby preferentially destroying the unmyelinated and ventrally located pain fibres. Approximately 10–12 lesions have to be placed in each spinal segment and multiple segments have to be treated for effective pain relief. The goal is to lesion only the dorsal roots, preserving the ventral ones.

The procedure is guided by motor evoked potentials and somatosensory evoked potentials to ensure no ventral roots are being affected and then stimulating each root to identify its functional value. The most common indication for this procedure is a brachial plexus avulsion injury. Others include cancer pain, cauda equina or spinal cord lesions, peripheral nerve lesions, and post-herpetic pain.

Extradural rhizotomies are quite similar to a ganglionectomy, however the ganglion is not resected. Using this technique, the corresponding motor root should be indentified and preserved whenever possible as it sometimes lies within the same dural encasement. Percutaneous radiofrequency rhizotomy or ganglionectomy may also be performed since unmyelinated or small myelinated neurons are sensitive to thermal lesioning. A tip electrode is placed within the neural foramen and 42 degrees Centigrade heat is passed for 15 seconds. A more permanent lesion may be performed by using 65–90 degrees of heat for 60–90 seconds.

Sympathectomy

Historically, sympathectomy was performed to treat epilepsy, glaucoma, goiter, spasticity, and even trigeminal neuralgia. In 1920 it was performed on a patient with hyperhidrosis yielding superior results and has become the most common indication for the procedure since. Other indications include sympathetically maintained pain and select cases of vasculitis. The characteristic sympathetic pain is severe, continuous and burning in nature with hyperalgesia and allodynia. Additionally, it may be accompanied by skin changes, temperature changes, and hyperhidrosis. Historically, this was described as reflex sympathetic dystrophy (RSD) but we now classify this painful disorder as complex regional pain syndrome (CRPS). Sympathetic blocks are the treatment of choice and the patient may show marked improvement in symptoms, but after repeated blocks, they tend to become less effective. At this point, sympathectomy is considered. For open surgery, supraclavicular, trans-axillary, and retroperitoneal flank approaches have all been described, but the most common route is the posterior paravertebral approach. For a thoracic sympathectomy, the procedure is performed in a prone or sitting position. The T2–3 costotransverse junction is exposed on the side of the pathology and it is removed along with the proximal 3 cm of the head of the ribs. Just deep to this, the sympathetic chain is visualized medial to the pleura, and using a clip, the chain is clipped above the T2 ganglion to include the inferior portion of the stellate ganglion, and below the T3 ganglion. Using sharp dissection, the chain is then cut between the clips. Rami communicantes adjacent to this are also clipped and cut to ensure a complete sympathectomy. In the case of thoracic sympathectomies, the procedure may also be performed thoracoscopically. Post-operative pneumothorax is a known complication and may require treatment with a chest tube, while Horner's syndrome may be caused by resecting the stellate ganglion and the fibers that innervate the papillary muscles. In the case of lumbar sympathectomies, a retroperitoneal approach is used. This is performed through a large flank incision carried down to the abdominal muscles, and, using blunt finger dissection, the peritoneum and renal tissue is displaced from the posterolateral abdominal wall. After identifying the quadrates lumborum, medial dissection exposes the psoas muscle and the vertebral bodies with the adjacent aorta if performed on the left, and vena cava if on the right. The lumbar sympathetic chain is then identified lying on the anterolateral part of the vertebral body between the psoas and aorta or vena cava. As described above, the L2 and L3 regions are clipped and cut along with the corresponding rami communicantes.

Hypophysectomy

In 1952, hypophysectomies were performed for palliation from intractable pain related to metastatic carcinoma. Treatment for this disease entity has evolved tremendously over the past decades, but widespread acceptance for hypophysectomies lasted over 30 years and the indications for such a procedure broadened. As a better understanding of hormones and their effect on cancers such as breast and prostate cancer developed, surgery to remove target hormone glands such as the ovaries, adrenal glands, or even part or all of the pituitary gland began in attempts to keep the patient's cancer at bay. The results of this were mixed and sometimes life threatening complications, such as addisonian crisis ensued in some cases, but a marked effect on pain relief was noticed. Open hypophysectomies transitioned to transsphenoidal approaches in the 1960s and this provided for a much less morbid surgical approach. Stereotactic radiofrequency and cryotherapy hypophysectomies were developed as well using radiographically guided instruments into the sella via a transsphenoidal approach. Though pain was usually only a secondary side effect of the procedure, patients continued to report immediate and long lasting pain relief after undergoing their surgery. Also in the 1960s, functional hypophysectomy for prostate carcinoma was attempted using brachytherapy with stereotactically implanted yttrium[90] with good pain relief. Additionally, in the late 1960s and 1970s stereotactic chemical ablation of the pituitary was performed with ethanol. It wasn't until the 1970's when the focus of reports on hypophysectomy focused primarily on pain relief and not the effect on tumor control. Fracchia et al reported on a series of 203 patients with advanced stage breast cancer treated with various forms of hypophysectomy, and 180 of 203 had pain relief with the procedure, although only 68 patients had no objective tumor response. The mechanism of pain control after hypophysectomy was initially viewed as a result of tumor shrinkage, and removing hormonal stimulation led to an overall decrease in size of the tumor burden, thereby causing less pain. As time passed, however, it was noticed that pain relief was achieved in non-hormone responsive tumors in the absence of clinical improvement. No identifiable pituitary hormone was known as a pain mediator, but it wasn't until 1984 that Ramirez and Levin suggested that the paraventricular nucleus (PVN) in the hypothalamus may be the key anatomic locus for pain control. Projections from the PVN are known to innervate the spinal dorsal horn, perimesencephalic gray, and other structures known to be important pain-modulating centers. Thus, the hypothalamus may in-fact be the key to the efficacy of hypophysectomy but it is only rarely performed today.

Midline Myelotomy

Interrupting ascending pathways that deliver nociceptive signals to the brain has been a mainstay of neurosurgical procedures aimed at the treatment of pain. Several of these procedures are prone to complications or necessitate bilateral procedures, and for this reason, the midline myelotomy was developed in 1926. The aim was to treat intractable visceral pelvic pain and the goal was to interrupt the crossing axons of the spinothalamic tract neurons on both sides by incising the midline of the posterior spinal cord. It was noted that pain relief was achieved at sites well distal to the levels of decussating axons. To this day, it is still unclear as to the mechanism of pain relief in midline myelotomies. Some proposed mechanisms include the pain relief is due to interruption of a polysynaptic pain pathway that ascends in the central gray of the spinal cord or a pain pathway that ascends near the midline of the posterior columns. Visceral pain pathways also ascend in the posterior columns and lesioning these crossed axons may also account for the success seen with midline myelotomies. The relief from this procedure is reported to last for 31 months after surgery without sensory, motor, or autonomic complications sometime seen with other procedures.

Anterolateral Cordotomy (AC)

The anterolateral quadrant of the spinal cord contains ascending pathways that are responsible for transmitting nociceptive information to the cerebral cortex. Of these, the most important are the lateral spinothalamic and spinoreticular tracts. These fibers project to the reticular formation and the thalamus respectively. The descending motor pathways in the lateral cortical-spinal tracts are located in the posterior quadrant of the cord along with the posterior columns, therefore pain can be relieved without loss of motor control or somesthetic and proprioceptive input. The procedure may be performed percutaneously or via open laminectomy.

The percutaneous procedure is performed with radiographic guidance by inserting a needle into the spinal cord via a lateral C1–C2 puncture. After penetration of the dura and prior to entering the cord, a small amount of dye is injected to outline the insertion of the dentate ligament. The radiofrequency needle is then inserted 3–4 mm into the anterior quadrant of the cord and a lesion created.

The open procedure may be performed unilaterally or bilaterally depending on the source of the patients pain but obviously is only valuable in abdominal and lower extremity pain. The patient is positioned prone and the spinous processes and lamina are removed at the T2–3 levels. The dura is then opened and the dentate ligament is cut to allow gentle rotation of the cord and visualization of the exiting ventral roots. Cutting the dentate ligament more superiorly and inferiorly may allow for more cord rotation. The pia over the anterolateral quadrant is then opened at an avascular area from the dentate ligament dorsally to the ventral root exit anteriorly. A cordotomy electrode is then inserted into the white matter and EMG activity can be evoked to ensure no corticospinal tract involvement. A blunt right angle probe that reflects the dimensions of that specific cord is then used to make the lesion. The probe is swept anteriorly avoiding the anterior spinal artery. Complications from AC are related to the tracts that are lesioned. Painful dysesthesias, decreased respiratory drive, bowel/bladder dysfunction, and sexual dysfunction, weakness, ataxia, and hypotension have all been reported, but overall AC can provide excellent short-term pain relief lasting 12–18 months. This makes it especially appropriate for patients with cancer pain.

Mesencephalotomy

Mesencephalotomy, or a lesion into the midbrain, was initially an extended cordotomy procedure intended to lesion the spinothalamic tract at the high level necessary to treat upper extremity pain or head and neck pain. Unfortunately, patients experienced very high rates of morbidity and mortality, and, if they survived the procedure, still had severe dysesthetic pain and a loss of sensation on the contralateral part of their body. Nevertheless, mesencephalotomy remains a consideration and treatment option for patient suffering from severe cancer pain, chronic pain, or central pain at locations too high to treat with an IT pump or anterolateral cordotomy. Extraocular palsy remains a known risk of this procedure and patients should be counseled on this prior to surgery. Today, the procedure has been modified to account for its prior morbidity, and involves lesioning the paleospinoreticular pathway. The mesencephalic reticular system actually lies between the spinothalamic tract and the central gray that surrounds the cerebral aqueduct where the pathways concerned with the emotional response to severe, intractable pain and the perception of suffering exist. In contrast, the spinothalamic tract is involved with perception of acute pain. Based on stimulation experiments, this newly discovered area lies medial to the spinothalamic tract and was involved with suffering and distress. As a result, the lesion was moved more medially to incorporate the lateral edge of the central gray and to include the medial part of the reticular formation. This procedure now actually spares the spinothalamic tract and provides bilateral pain relief. Additionally, it has been shown that intrinsic chemical changes occur as a result of severe pain and emotional distress, and these changes can be demonstrated on a neural level. Therefore, the goal of mesencephalotomy is accomplished by modifying the perception of pain itself.

The procedure itself is carried out using stereotactic MRI guidance and electrode insertion into the mesencephalic spinoreticular tract avoiding the tectum. Intra-operative stimulation is used to verify location of the lesion site between 5 and 300 Hz. At the target site, a small radiofrequency lesion is made which usually produces a severe emotional response and a feeling of pain relief at the core of the body. If the electrode is too lateral, in the spinothalamic tract, paresthesias on the contralateral body are felt. If the electrode is too close to the medial lemniscus, contralateral tremor is seen.

Medial Thalamotomy (MT)

The spinothalamic tract terminates in the medial thalamus, and it has, therefore, been postulated that lesioning the medial thalamus might alleviate chronic and severe pain. Further proof that the medial thalamus is involved in nociceptive processing is that abnormal electrical activity is observed here in patients suffering from chronic pain. Based on electrical recordings, it has been shown that the most intense bursting of activity is in cells located in the posterior aspect of the core of the ventrocaudal nucleus and in the posteroinferior area. It is in these areas that the spinothalamic tract terminations are most dense. MT was actually the first stereotactic brain operation for pain performed. Given that these areas of the thalamus are the recipient of spinothalamic tract fibers and the main pain processing center, MT has been used to treat somatic, deafferentation, and central pain. In the medial tier of thalamic nuclei lies the centralis lateralis (CL), a nucleus packed densely with spinothalamic tract terminals. The centromedian and parafascicularis nuclei are other neighboring intralaminar structures of the thalamus that receive a much less dense concentration of spinothalamic tract projections. These nuclei then collectively project to cortical structures and the striatum. Pre-operative determination of lesion location is made by stereotactic MRI or CT. Surgical lesioning of the medial thalamus is then made anatomically, based on calculated positions from the anterior commisure-posterior commisure (AC–PC) lines, and physiologically, based on spontaneous or evoked electrical activity. The most common medial thalamus lesion is made in the centromedian and parafascicularis. Lesions may be placed unilaterally or bilaterally. Pain relief effects are initially quite good but tend to decrease with time and can recur. It is for this reason that malignant pain has been shown to have a much better treatment result after MT as compared to central or neurogenic pain. Complications rates for MT are low and mostly due to lesions extending into the lateral thalamus resulting in severe dysesthesias.

Cingulotomy

A cingulotomy refers to ablation of the anterior cingulate gyrus which includes both the cortical regions and the subcortical regions, namely the cingulum fasciculus, a major association tract of the limbic system located in the white matter underneath the cingulate gyrus cortex. Most surgical procedures for pain have aimed at disrupting the neural pathways conveying a painful stimulus, often at the expense of normal somatic sensation. The cingulotomy procedure, however, has no influence on somatic nociception. It is thought to produce pain relief by altering the patient's emotional reaction to pain and by increasing the tolerance to the subjective and emotional feelings of pain. No afferent pain pathways are actually lesioned here, as the affective components such as fear, depression, and suffering are the real target of therapy. Cingulotomy has therefore become indicated in patients with affective disorders suffering from chronic pain. Cancer pain, as well as various nonmalignant types of pain with a psychogenic element, has also been treated with cingulotomy. Cingulotomy should only be considered in patients suffering from persistent, debilitating, and treatment refractory pain. The mechanism of a cingulotomy is thought to involve the complex fiber pathway that receives and transmits signals to both the limbic and extra-limbic structures in the vicinity of the cingulum. As with other stereotactic lesioning procedures, it is performed under local anesthesia with intravenous sedation and targets are chosen on pre-operative MRI (Figure 5.2). Coordinates are calculated for a point in the anterior cingulated gyrus 2–2.5 cm posterior to the tip of the frontal horn of the lateral ventricle, 7 mm from the midline, and 1–2 mm above the roof of the lateral ventricles. The lesions are produced using a thermocoupled

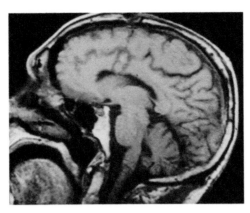

FIGURE 5.2   Sagittal T1 weighted MRI of anterior cingulotomy lesion <48 hours after surgery with dramatic pain relief in a 47 year old woman with diffuse osseous metastases.

coagulation electrode measuring 10 mm in length and 1.6 mm in diameter inserted to the target points. Lesions are created by heating the electrode tip to 85°C for 90 seconds. After the electrode tip has cooled, it may be withdrawn and the procedure repeated bilaterally. Complications are relatively few but can involve temporary bladder retention or incontinence, isolated seizures, hemorrhage, or unsteady gait. About 25–40% of patients will require repeat cingulotomy with an attempt to lesion more of the cingulum fasciculus.

Success with this surgery seems to surround the volume of damaged cingulum fasciculus, for best results, bilateral cingulotomies should be performed. Long-term follow up and adequate pain recording diaries are crucial for these patients and, again noted was the inverse relationship between pain-free patients and survival.

Further Reading

1. Burgess PR, Perl ER. Myelinated afferent fibers responding specifically to noxious stimulation of the skin. *J Physiol (Lond.)*. 1967;190:541–562.
2. Koerber HR, et al. Properties of somata of spinal dorsal root ganglion cells differ according to peripheral receptor innervated. *J Neurophysiol*. 1988;60:1584–1596.
3. Treede RD, et al. The cortical representation of pain. *Pain*. 1999;79:105–111.
4. Hardy JD, Wolff HG, Goodell H. *Pain Sensations and Reactions*. Baltimoer, Md: Williams and Wilkins; 1952.
5. Loeser JD, Sears JL, Newman RI. Interdisciplinary, multimodal management of chronic pain. In: Bonica JJ, ed. *The Management of Pain*. Philadelphia: Lea and Febinger; 1990. p. 2107–2120.
6. Wall PD, Sweet WH. Temporary abolition of pain in man. *Science*. 1967;155:108–109.
7. Sweet WH, Wepsic JG. Treatment of chronic pain by stimulation of fibers of primary afferent neurons. *Trans Am Neurol Assoc*. 1968;93:103–107.
8. Racz GB, Browne T, Lewis Jr. R. Peripheral stimulator implant for treatment of causalgia caused by electrical burns. *Tex Med*. 1988;84:45–50.

9. Melzack R, Wall PD. Pain mechanisms: a new theory. *Science*. 1965;150:971–979.
10. Ignelzi RJ, Nyquist JV. Direct effect of electrical stimulation on peripheral nerve evoked activity: implications in pain relief. *J Neurosurg*. 1976;45:159–165.
11. Mannheimer C, et al. Epidural spinal electrical stimulation in severe angina pectoris. *Br Heart J*. 1988;59:56–61.
12. Jessurun GAJ, et al. Current views on neurostimulation in the treatment of cardiac ischemic syndromes. *Pain*. 1996;66:109–116.
13. Tasker RR. Deafferentation. In: Wall PD, Melzack R, eds. *Textbook of Pain*. Edinburgh: Churchill Livingstone; 1984. p. 119–132.
14. Pagni CA. Central pain due to spinal cord and brain stem damage. In: Wall PD, Melzack R, eds. *Textbook of Pain*. Edinburgh: Churchill Livingstone; 1984. p. 481–495.
15. Yamamoto T, et al. Pharmacological classification of central post stroke pain: comparison with the results of chronic motor cortex stimulation therapy. *Pain*. 1997;72:5–12.
16. Tsubokawa T, et al. Chronic motor cortex stimulation for treatment of central pain. *Acta Neurochir*. 1991;52(suppl):137–139.
17. Tsubokawa T, et al. Chronic motor cortex stimulation in patients with thalamic pain. *J Neurosurg*. 1993;78:393–401.
18. Burchiel K. *Surgical Management of Pain*. New York: Thieme Medical Publishers; 2002. p. 565–576.
19. Heath R. *Studies in Schizophrenia: A Multidisciplinary Approach to Mind-Brain Relationship*. Cambridge, Ma: Harvard University Press; 1954.
20. Richardson DE, Akil H. Pain reduction by electrical brain stimulation in man, part 1: acute administration in periaqueductal and periventricular sites. *J Neurosurg*. 1977;47:178–183.
21. Richardson DE, Akil H. Pain reduction by electrical brain stimulation in man, part 2: chronic self-administration in the periventricular gray matter. *J Neurosurg*. 1977;47:184–194.
22. Adams JE, Hosobuchi Y, Fields HL. Stimulation of internal capsule for relief of chronic pain. *J Neurosurg*. 1974;41:740–744.
23. Reynolds D. Surgery in the rat during electrical analgesia induced by focal brain stimulation. *Science*. 1969;164:444–445.
24. Richardson DE, Akil H. Long term results of periventricular gray self-stimulation. *Neurosurgery*. 1977;1:199–202.
25. Young RF, Kroening R, Fulton W, et al. Electrical stimulation of the brain in treatment of chronic pain. *J Neurosurg*. 1985;62:289–396.
26. Dieckmann G, Witzmann A. Initial and long-term results of deep brain stimulation for chronic intractable pain. *Appl Neurophysiol*. 1982;45:167–172.
27. Kumar K, Toth C, Nath RK. Deep brain stimulation for intractable pain: a 15 year experience. *Neurosurgery*. 1997;40:736–747.
28. Levy RM, Lamb S, Adams JE. Treatment of chronic pain by deep brain stimulation: long-term follow up and review of the literature. *Neurosurgery*. 1987;21:885–893.
29. Schaltenbrand G, Wahren E. *Atlas for Stereotaxy of the Human Brain*. New York: George Thieme Verlag; 1977.
30. *The use of opioids for the treatment of chronic pain. A consensus statement from the American Academy of Pain Medicine and the American Pain Society*. Glenview, Il. American Academy of Pain Medicine and American Pain Society; 1997.
31. Paice JA, Penn RD, Shott S. Intraspinal morphine for chronic pain: a retrospective, multicenter study. *J Pain Symptom Manage*. 1996;11:71–80.
32. Winkelmuller M, Winkelmuller W. Long-term effects of continuous intrathecal opioid treatment in chronic pain of nonmalignant etiology. *J Neurosurg*. 1996;85:458–467.
33. Mackinnon SE, Dellon AL. *Surgery of the Peripheral Nerve*. New York: Thieme Medical Publishers; 1988.
34. Coggeshall RE. Afferent fibers in the ventral root. *Neurosurgery*. 1979;4:443–448.

35. Young RF. Dorsal rhizotomy and dorsal root ganglionectomy. In: Youmans JR, ed. *Neurological Surgery* (4th ed.). Philadelphia: WB Saunders; 1996. p. 3442–3451.

36. Drott C. The history of cervicothoracic sympathectomy. *Eur J Surg Suppl.* 1994;572:5–7.

37. Kotzareff A. Resection partielle de trone sympathetique cervical droit pour hyperhidrose unilateral. *Rev Med Suisse Romande.* 1920;40:111–113.

38. Sindou M, Quoex C, Baleydier C. Fiber organization at the posterior spinal cord-rootlet junction in man. *J Comp Neurol.* 1974;153:15–26.

39. Sindou M. *Etude De La Junction Radiculo-Medullaire Posterieure: La Radicellotomie Posterieure Selective Dans La Chirurgie De La Douleur.* Lyon: These med. 1972;182.

40. Nashold BS, Ostdahl PH. Dorsal root entry zone lesions for pain relief. *J Neurosurg.* 1979;51:59–69.

41. Burchiel K. *Surgical Management of Pain.* New York: Thieme Medical Publishers; 2002. p. 701–713.

42. White JC, Sweet WH. *Pain and the Neurosurgeon: A Forty Year Experience.* Springfield, IL: Charles C. Thomas; 1969.

43. Gybels JM, Sweet WH. *Neurosurgical Treatment of Persistent Pain: Physiological and Pathological Mechanisms of Human Pain.* Basel: Karger; 1989.

44. Nauta HJW, Hewitt E, Westlund KN, Willis WD. Surgical interruption of a midline dorsal column visceral pain pathway. *J Neurosurg.* 1997;86:538–542.

45. King RB. Anterior commissurotomy for intractable pain. *J Neurosurg.* 1977;47:7–11.

46. Hitchcock E. Stereotaxic cervical myelotomy. *J Neurol Neurosurg Psychiatry.* 1970;33:224–230.

47. Schvarcz JR. Spinal cord stereotactic techniques re trigeminal nucleotomy and extralemniscal myelotomy. *Appl Neurophysiol.* 1978;41:99–112.

48. Smith MV, Apkarian AV, Hodge CJ. Somatosensory response properties of contralaterally projecting spinothalamic and nonspinothalamic neurons in the second cervical segment of the cat. *J Neurophysiol.* 1991;66:83–102.

49. Hodge Jr CJ, Apkarian AV. The spinothalamic tract. *Crit Rev Neurobiol.* 1990;5:363–397.

50. Willis WD. The origin and destination of pathways involved in pain transmission. In: Wall PD, Melzack R, eds. *Textbook of Pain.* New York, NY: Churchill Livingstone; 1984. p. 88–99.

51. Krieger AJ, Rosomoff HL. Sleep-induced apnea. 1. A respiratory and autonomic dysfunction syndrome following bilateral percutaneous cervical cordotomy. *J Neurosurg.* 1974;40:168–180.

52. Nathan PW, Smith MC. The centrifugal pathway for micturition within the spinal cord. *J Neurol Neurosurg Psychiatry.* 1958;21:177–189.

53. Perrault M, et al. L'hypophysectomie totale dans le traitment du cancer du sien: premier cas francais: avenir de la method. *Therapie.* 1952;7:290–300.

54. Scott WW. Endocrine management of disseminated prostatic cancer, including bilateral adrenalectomy and hypophysectomy. *Trans Am Assoc Genitourinary Surg.* 1952;44:101–104.

55. Huggins C, Berganstal DM. Inhibition of human mammary and prostatic cancers by adrenalectomy. *Cancer Res.* 1952;12:134–141.

56. Kennedy BJ, French LA, Peyton WT. Hypophysectomy in advanced breast cancer. *N Engl J Med.* 1956;255:1165–1172.

57. Talairach J, Tournoux P. Appareil de stereotaxie hypophysaire pour voie d'abord nasale. *Neurochirurgie.* 1955;1:127–131.

58. Fergusson JD, Phillips DE. A clinical evaluation of radioactive pituitary implantation in the treatment of advanced carcinoma of the prostate. *Br J Urol.* 1962;34:485–492.

59. Morrica G. Chemical hypophysectomy for cancer pain. In: Bonica JJ, editor. *Advances in Neurology,* Vol. 4. New York: Raven Press; 1974. p. 707–714.

60. Fracchia AA, Farrow JH, Miller TR, Tollefson RH, Greenberg EJ, Knapper WH. Hypophysectomy as compared with adrenalectomy in the treatment of advanced carcinoma of the breast. *Surg Gynecol Obstet.* 1971;133:241–246.

61. Ramirez LF, Levin AB. Pain relief after hypophysectomy. *Neurosurgery.* 1984;14:499–504.

62. Levin AB, Ramirez LF, Katz J. The use of stereotaxic chemical hypophysectomy in the treatment of thalamic pain syndrome. *J Neurosurg.* 1983;59:1002–1006.

63. Nashold Jr. BS. Brainstem stereotaxic procedures. In: Schaltenbrand G, Walker AE, eds. *Stereotaxy of the Human Brain.* New York: Georg Thieme Verlag; 1982. p. 475–483.

64. Bowsher D. Termination of the central pain pathway in man: the conscious appreciation of pain. *Brain.* 1957;80:606–622.

65. Mehler WR. The anatomy of the so called "pain tract" in man: an analysis of the course and distribution of the ascending fibers of the fasciculus anterolateralis. In: French JD, Porter RW, eds. *Basic Research in Paraplegia.* Springfield, IL: Charles C. Thomas; 1962. p. 26–55.

66. Mehler WR. Further notes on the centre median nucleus of Luys. In: Purpura DP, Yahr MD, eds. *The Thalamus.* New York: Columbia University Press; 1966. p. 109–127.

67. Walker AE. The thalamus of the chimpanzee. I. Terminations of the somatic afferent systems. *Cong INIA Neurol.* 1938;1:99–127.

68. Spiegel EA, Wycis HT. *Stereoencephalotomy, Part II, Clinical and Physiological Applications.* New York: Grune & Stratton; 1962.

69. Jeanmonod D, Magnin M, Morel A. Thalamus and neurogenic pain: physiological, anatomical, and clinical data. *Neuroreport.* 1993;4:475–478.

70. Foltz EL, White LE. Pain relief by frontal cingulomotomy. *J Neurosurg.* 1962;19:89–100.

71. Freeman W, Watts JW. Pain of organic disease relieved by prefrontal lobotomy. *Lancet.* 1946;1:953–955.

72. Foltz EL, White LE. The role of rostral cingulumotomy in pain relief. *Int J Neurol.* 1968;6:353–373.

73. Foltz EL. Current status and the use of rostral cingulumotomy. *South Med J.* 1968;61:899–908.

74. Ballantine Jr HT, Cosgrove GR, Giriunas IE. Surgical treatment of intractable psychiatric illness and chronic pain by cingulotomy. In: Schmidek HH, Sweet WH, eds. *Operative Neurosurgical Techniques: Indications, Methods, and Results.* Philadelphia: WB Saunders; 1995. p. 1423–1430.

75. Hurt RW, Ballantine Jr. HT. Stereotactic anterior cingulated lesions for persistent pain: a report of 68 cases. *Clin Neurosurg.* 1974;21:334–351.

6

Thalamocortical Abnormalities in Spinal Cord Injury Pain

Asaf Keller[1] and Radi Al-Masri[2]

[1]Department of Anatomy and Neurobiology, University of Maryland School of Medicine, Baltimore, MD, USA, [2]Department of Endodontics, Prosthodontics and Operative Dentistry, Baltimore College of Dental Surgery, University of Maryland Baltimore, Baltimore, Maryland, USA

SCI-PAIN

More than a million Americans live with the consequence of spinal cord injury (SCI). SCI is a leading cause of paralysis, and may lead to other catastrophic consequences, including compromised bladder and bowel functions,[1] emotional and psychological distress[2] and loss of sexual function.[3]

SCI results not only in debilitating motor, sensory and cognitive deficits, but also in chronic, excruciating and relentless pain (SCI-Pain). SCI-Pain may involve a restricted part of the body, such as a hand, but it commonly involves extensive body regions.[4] Patients often describe more than one pain quality, including burning pain (most common), aching, and pressing pain.[5–7] The pain is unrelenting, and has been described "as if knives heated in Hell's hottest corner were tearing me to pieces."[8] This unremitting pain can be diffuse, bilateral, and often extends to locations caudal to the spinal injury ("below-lesion").[9–11] Perhaps most debilitating—and puzzling—is the presence, in nearly all patients, of chronic, spontaneous pain.[4,12,13] SCI-pain is usually resistant to treatment.[14]

In most SCI patients chronic pain first appears more than one year after the injury.[15–17] The latent period between the spinal injury and the development of chronic pain offers clues as to the pathophysiology of SCI-Pain. This latent period also provides *a window of opportunity* for interventions to prevent or minimize the development of SCI-Pain. The delayed expression of SCI-Pain, the diffuse localization of painful symptoms, and the presence of pain below the denervated spinal segment strongly suggest the occurrence of maladaptive plasticity not only in the spinal cord, but also in supraspinal structures.[18]

Pain resulting from SCI is related to central pain syndrome (CPS), defined as "pain initiated or caused by a primary lesion or dysfunction in the central nervous system".[19] CPS results from a variety of conditions and insults at any level of the spinal cord and the brain. The most common conditions are cerebrovascular accidents (strokes), SCI and multiple sclerosis. The prevalence of pain in these conditions is alarmingly high: As many as 60 to 80% of SCI patients experience pain, with at least ⅓ of the patients rating the pain as severe.[4,11,20–25] Almost 30% of multiple sclerosis patients develop chronic neuropathic pain, and in stroke patients the prevalence is at least 10%.[4,11,20] As discussed below, a common pathophysiology—central sensitization—might underlie neuropathic pain in these different conditions.

ANIMAL MODELS OF SCI-PAIN

Several animal models have been developed to study the pathophysiology of SCI-Pain (Table 6.1). Some models use controlled spinal contusions to mimic clinically relevant traumatic injuries.[30,32,33] Others have used ischemic lesions,[39] spinal injections of neurotoxins,[36,37] cuts that sever the spinal cord (hemisection)[34,35] or localized cuts in the spinal cord (cordotomy).[27,28] Most of these models rely on measures of evoked pain and hypersensitivity, such as mechanical and thermal withdrawal thresholds, to assess hyperalgesia or allodynia. However, they rarely attempt to quantify *spontaneous pain*, which is the single most common and debilitating complaint of SCI patients.[10,20,44] Further, in many of these models, animals develop complications from injury that can confound pain testing, such as movement deficits or paralysis, and infection. Movement deficits, in particular, complicate attempts to quantify pain by measuring withdrawal latency or threshold, as these metrics assume intact motor functions.

We have adapted and refined a rodent model of SCI-Pain.[42,43,45,46] Because the spinothalamic system is affected in all SCI-Pain patients (see below), we produce electrolytic lesions that include the spinothalamic tract. An important advantage of this model is that it spares motor functions, allowing us to use paw-withdrawal as a metric for responses to noxious stimuli. In every case in which lesions affected the integrity of the spinothalamic tract, animals developed significant hyperalgesia, evidenced as increased responsiveness to mechanical or thermal stimuli.[45]

TABLE 6.1 Animal Models of Spinal Cord Injury Pain

Model	Species	Method	Behavioral Findings	Characteristics
Anterolateral cut model[26-28]	Monkey, rat	Anterolateral cut of the spinal cord to interrupt the STT	Over grooming and below-level bilateral hyperalgesia to electrical and mechanical stimulation	• Injury to the STT which is thought to be necessary for the development of central pain • Well characterized behaviorally
Contusion model[29-33]	Rat	Applying a defined force using an impact probe or by dropping of a weight on the dorsal aspect of the spinal cord	Eighty percent of animals develop at-level and above-level mechanical and thermal hyperalgesia	• Mimics clinical injury • Associated with large variability in extent of lesion and pathophysiological consequences • evaluating below level pain complicated because hindlimbs are profoundly affected by lesion • Electrophysiological and molecular consequences are well characterized
Hemisection model[34,35]	Rat	Unilateral cut of the spinal cord at the mid thoracic level	All animals develop bilateral below and above-level bilateral mechanical and thermal hyperalgesia	• Extensive cut to the spinal cord • Offers little advantage over the anterolateral section model
Quisqualate model[36,37]	Rat	Injection of neurotoxic chemicals into the dorsal horn	Fifty percent of the animals develop over grooming in areas somatotopically related to the lesion and at and below-level mechanical hyperalgesia	• High variability in extent of lesion and behavioral consequences

(Continued)

TABLE 6.1 (Continued)

Model	Species	Method	Behavioral Findings	Characteristics
Ischemia model[38,39]	Rat	Injecting a photo sensitive dye through circulation and using a focus a laser beam to region of the spinal cord. The interaction of the laser beam with the photosensitive dye results in a to lesion the gray matter of the spinal cord	Forty four percent of animals develop at-level and below level mechanical allodynia. None of the animals develop thermal hyperalgesia	• High variability in extent of lesion and behavioral consequences
Discrete avulsion of dorsal roots[40]	Rat	Unilateral avulsion of T13 and L1 dorsal root damaging Lissauer's tract, dorsal horn and dorsal column	Bilateral below-level mechanical hyperalgesia	• Localized injury to the dorsal horn • Injury is not limited to the central nervous system
Electrolytic lesions model[41–43]	Rat	Localized electrolytic lesions of the anterolateral quadrant of the spinal cord	Ninety four percent of animals develop bilateral below and above-level mechanical and thermal hyperalgesia	• Discrete localized lesion in the STT • Low morbidity and no loss of function following surgery

Significantly, and consistent with the human condition, hyperalgesia in rats develops after a latent period of two to three weeks, and never reverses.[45]

We recognized that the well-established metrics to assess hyperalgesia are limited in that they rely on reflexive measures—latency or thresholds of responses to noxious mechanical or thermal stimuli. Further, these methods cannot assess the main complaint in humans with SCI-Pain—the presence of spontaneous pain. This is a limitation inherent to all animal models of pain.[47] To obviate this shortcoming we adapted and modified a conditioned place preference paradigm[48] to test if animals with SCI develop signs consistent with spontaneous pain.[49] This paradigm relies on the fact that pain relief is rewarding to animals. Rats with spinal cord lesions and sham-operated controls are habituated to a two-chamber, conditioned place preference box, and the time spent in each chamber is recorded. Rats then undergo a three-day conditioning phase in which they receive intra-ventricular clonidine infusion as an analgesic. The following day they are again permitted to move freely between the chambers to determine if the treatment changed their preference for one of the chambers. We found that clonidine was rewarding to animals with SCI, but not to sham operated controls.[49] We find also that replacing clonidine injections with stimulation of the motor cortex—discussed later in this chapter as a potential therapy for SCI-Pain—results also in a development of preference for the chamber in which treatment is delivered.[49] These findings are consistent with the conclusion that animals with SCI suffer from "spontaneous pain."

Taken together, these findings demonstrate that our model of central pain recapitulates key clinical characteristics of SCI-Pain. This model allowed us to directly investigate the mechanisms responsible for SCI-Pain. Importantly, we have recently confirmed that both the behavioral and electrophysiological deficits induced by these electrolytic lesions occur also after contusion injury to the spinal cord, a pathology more similar to SCI in humans (C. Raver, J. Wu., A. Faden and A.K., unpublished observations). This confirms that the electrolytic lesion model produces pain related pathologies that are relevant to the human condition. These findings suggest that this model can be used to study the pathophysiology of SCI-Pain.

PATHOPHYSIOLOGY OF SCI-PAIN

Since the first published description of central pain, nearly 130 years ago,[50,51] several hypotheses have been proposed to explain its pathophysiology.[4,11,52,53] Many were disproved with time, and many remain controversial. Fortunately—and despite the clinical variability in presentation and variability in size, location and causes of SCI—there is general agreement on a number of pathophysiological factors.

Many of the earliest reported cases of central pain were based on pain caused by damage or injury to the thalamus.[50,54,55] As a result, thalamic abnormalities were thought to be required for development of pain and the condition was referred to for decades by the misleading term "thalamic pain." It is now established that central pain can result from damage to any structure along the afferent spino-thalamo-cortical pathway that conveys pain and temperature information.[4,56–60] This pathway includes the spinothalamic tract (STT) in the spinal cord and brainstem; thalamic nuclei that receive STT input, including the posterior thalamus (PO), the mediodorsal thalamus (MD) and the ventroposterior (ventrobasal) complex (VP), the internal capsule, and cortical areas such as the primary (SI) and second (S2) somatosensory cortex.[61]

For SCI-Pain to develop, the insult must involve the STT that conveys pain and temperature information. Indeed, there are no documented cases of SCI-Pain after lesions that spare the tract, such as lesions involving only the dorsal column-medial lemniscal pathway.[52,62] Consistent with an obligatory role for the STT is the finding that essentially all central pain patients have altered pain and temperature sensation, while abnormalities of tactile sensation occur in only a subset of patients.[4,56,63]

SPINAL ABNORMALITIES

As expected, SCI-Pain is associated with widespread changes in the spinal cord, beginning both immediately and progressing, at variable delays, after the spinal injury. These maladpative changes include ischemia, necrosis, deafferentation, anatomical and synaptic plasticity of spinal circuits, abnormal expression of channels and receptors on spinal neurons and glia, changes in cell-signaling pathways and activation of glia.[35,64–70] Changes in the bulbo-spinal descending pain modulatory system might also contribute to SCI-Pain.[69,71]

However, surgical interventions that disconnect affected spinal segments from the brain—including cordotomy, cordectomy, myelotomy, and dorsal root entry zone lesion—have limited, if any, efficacy in treating SCI-Pain.[65,72,73] Further, the delayed expression of SCI-Pain and the diffuse localization of painful symptoms suggest that the pathophysiology involves more than just the direct effects at the denervated spinal segments. Rather, these features of SCI-Pain strongly suggest the fundamental involvement of maladaptive plasticity in *supraspinal structures* where inputs from various body parts converge.

Consistent with this notion, it has been shown repeatedly that SCI is associated with neuronal hyperexcitability and changes in glial activation in the thalamus.[30,43,70,74,75] The mechanism by which these central maladaptive changes occur are only now being understood.

THALAMIC ABNORMALITIES

One hypothesis that remains in favor, almost a century since it was first formulated, is that CPS—including SCI-Pain—results from abnormally suppressed inhibition in the thalamus.[55] However, the site of operation of this disinhibition remains unknown.[4,52] It has been argued that the medial lemniscal pathway normally inhibits the spinothalamic system, and that this inhibition is suppressed in CPS conditions. Alternatively, it has been proposed that either descending cortical inputs or ascending spinal inputs to the thalamus are involved in this disinhibition.[55,76] A more recent elaboration of the Head and Holmes hypothesis[55] posits that the disinhibition results from a loss of the discriminative thermosensory representation in the central nervous system.[77] This "thermosensory disinhibition hypothesis" assumes that pain is relayed from the spinal cord through independent thalamic pain/temperature nuclei that serve as specific relays in the ascending pain system. This viewpoint stands in contrast to descriptions of more widespread distributions of STT fibers,[78,79] and is inconsistent with clinical findings implicating other thalamic nuclei in SCI-Pain[58,80]

These controversies notwithstanding, thalamic changes have been associated with pain after SCI in humans,[81,82] primates[83] and rats.[43,45,84,85] Unfortunately, the consensus appears to end there, as there are conflicting hypotheses regarding the specific thalamic nuclei involved and the underlying mechanisms responsible for altered function.[4,52]

Abnormalities in VPL

It is natural that the ventrobasal (or, ventroposterior) nucleus of the thalamus attracts attention as a likely mediator of SCI-Pain. It is considered the "specific", or, first-order somatosensory thalamic nucleus,[86] and it receives converging spinal inputs from the dorsal columns and the spinothalamic tract.[61,87–89] Both animal and human studies suggest that SCI-Pain is correlated with changes in this nucleus.[69] Most studies have focused on the lateral segment of the ventroposterior nucleus (VPL) because this is where noxious and innocuous inputs from the limbs and trunk are processed (the medial segment, VPM, processes inputs from the head and neck). Results from animal studies, using various models of SCI, support a temporal correlation between the slow time-course of development of SCI-Pain (see above) and the activation of chemokines, microglia and unique sodium channels.[70,90] Of particular interest are studies by Hains, Saab, Waxman and collaborators, demonstrating that after SCI, there occurs in VPL neurons (as well as in spinal neurons) an abnormal expression of $Na_v1.3$, a rapidly re-priming voltage dependent sodium channel.[91–93] The appearance of this channel is thought to be responsible, at least in part, for the hyper-excitability of VPL neurons after SCI, reported by several groups (e.g.[43,94]). The hyper-excitability is expressed both as an increase in the spontaneous firing rate of VPL neurons, and in their increased responsiveness to sensory stimuli, compared to responses of neurons from sham or naïve animals. A causal relationship between the expression of $Na_v1.3$ in VPL and SCI-Pain is supported by findings that both the signs of pain (hyperalgesia) and the abnormal activity of VPL neurons can be reversed by $Na_v1.3$ antisense.[91]

The Role of Thalamic Bursts

In addition to the increase in spontaneous and evoked firing described above, VPL neurons from SCI animals—as well as in its homologue in some human studies—have been reported to display an abnormally high incidence of "bursting activity".[27,43,74,91,95,96] However, the causal relationship between the expression of these bursts and the perception of pain has been questioned (reviewed in Dostrovsky[97]). For example, burst activity occurs in the thalamus of both individuals suffering from chronic pain and in pain-free patients.[98,99] Further, stimulating the thalamus of humans with burst patterns fails to elicit pain.[99]

It is possible that the controversy regarding the role of thalamic bursts in pain perception is a semantic one. The original definition of a burst usually refers to calcium-dependent spike bursts, characterized in thalamic neurons through intracellular recordings.[100] In extracellular recordings it is difficult to distinguish calcium-dependent bursts from epochs of high frequency firing of "conventional" sodium spikes, and most studies do not make that distinction. Thus, it is not possible to determine, from previous studies, whether the reported increases in "bursts" are simply a reflection of increased firing rates, or whether they truly represent a calcium-dependent phenomenon. We return to this issue below, when describing our data on burst firing in other thalamic nuclei.

Abnormalities in Higher Order Thalamic Nuclei

Pain is a multi-dimensional experience, including components such as sensory-discriminative, affective-motivational and cognitive-evaluative.[101–103] These components are subserved by a "pain neuromatrix", comprised of a distributed neuronal network that includes somatosensory, limbic and other structures.[104,105] Some have suggested that the different dimensions of pain experience arise from activity in different components of this matrix.[106,107] For example, the "lateral system," including VP and the primary somatosensory cortex, was proposed to be involved primarily in the sensory-discrimintive dimension of pain. The "medial system"— including the posterior thalamic nucleus (PO) and medial thalamic nuclei such as mediodorsal (MD), and the anterior cingulate and the prefrontal cortex—is thought to be involved primarily in the affective-motivational dimensions of pain (but see, e.g. Bushnell et al.[108]).

There are indications that the symptoms of CPS preferentially activate components of the affective medial system.[102,104,109–111] We therefore asked whether SCI-Pain is associated with abnormalities in thalamic nuclei associated with the medial system, the PO and MD nuclei.

Posterior Nucleus of the Thalamus

The posterior nucleus (PO) in rodents is a higher-order somatosensory thalamic nucleus important for processing both innocuous and noxious sensory information and relaying these signals to the cortex. Its analogs in primates, including humans, are thought to include the thalamic posterior complex and the anterior pulvinar.[61,112] PO receives dense ascending projections from the spinothalamic and the trigeminothalamic tracts.[113–121] More specifically, both lamina I and deeper layers of the spinal and medullary dorsal horns project to PO in monkeys and rats.[115,122,123] In addition, PO receives input from the deep layers of the superior colliculus[124,125] as well as from the zona incerta (discussed below)[126,127] and the anterior pretectal nucleus.[128–130] PO also receives input from, and sends reciprocal projections to, the primary somatosensory cortex (SI) and the second somatosensory cortex (SII).[131–135] The posterior portion of PO projects also to limbic areas such as the insular cortex and the amygdala.[115,136]

Pioneering studies by Poggio and Mountcastle in the anesthetized cat revealed that PO responds preferentially to noxious peripheral stimulation, such as cuts or pinpricks. Neurons in this region have relatively large receptive fields that are often bilateral.[137] Later, very similar findings were reported by others studying anesthetized and unanesthetized cats and monkeys,[138–145] indicating that neurons in PO are involved in processing noxious information.

Together with the dense ascending input from spinal pathways that convey noxious information, the cortical projections to both SI and SII, and the projections to areas of the limbic circuit, these data suggest that the posterior thalamus plays an important role in normal pain processing and identify it as a target that may be affected in conditions of chronic pain. We therefore compared neuronal activity in the PO thalamus of rats with experimental SCI-Pain (using our model described above; similar changes occur after contusion-SCI) with that in sham-operated rats.[45]

We recorded spontaneous and stimulus-evoked activity in the two main somatosensory thalamic clusters: the "first-order" ventroposterior complex and the "higher-order" PO nucleus.[146] Spontaneous firing of ventroposterior thalamic neurons was about 4-fold higher in SCI-Pain rats, compared to controls, consistent with other reports described above. Stimulus-evoked responses remained unchanged in this nucleus. By contrast, spontaneous firing of PO neurons in SCI-Pain rats **increased 30-fold**, and their responses to peripheral stimuli were also significantly higher than in shams. These findings strongly implicate PO as a site of maladaptive plasticity in SCI-Pain.

We describe above the controversy related to the causal role of burst firing in the pathogenesis of SCI-Pain. In our study of PO neurons in animals with SCI,[45] we defined bursts of action potentials recorded extracellularly as clusters of at least three spikes, with inter-spike intervals of ≤ 4 ms, in which the first spike in the burst has a preceding inter-spike interval of ≥ 100 ms. This definition is based on previous intracellular studies of bursting in thalamic nuclei.[147–149] Using these criteria, and comparing to PO neurons from sham-operated controls, in PO neurons from SCI rats we found no significant difference in either the percentage of spontaneously bursting cells or in the frequency of spontaneous bursts. Similarly, neither the percentage of cells that burst in response to sensory stimuli, nor the incidence of evoked bursts were significantly different in rats with SCI. These findings indicate that the incidence of spike bursts—as defined in this study—remain unchanged in PO neurons. Thus these findings do not resolve the current controversy regarding the causal role of spike bursts in CPS.[97]

Mediodorsal Thalamus

Like PO, the mediodorsal thalamus (MD) is a "higher-order" thalamic nucleus that receives direct input from the STT[150–153] and from zona incerta.[154,155] MD is reciprocally connected with several areas of the limbic circuit, including the anterior cingulate cortex, the insular cortex, and the amygdala.[156–164] In addition, MD receives inputs from diverse structures, including the olfactory bulb,[165,166] substantia nigra,[167] superior colliculus,[168] and hypothalamus.[169]

In rodents, MD can be divided into three regions, the medial, central and lateral. The divisions and cortical projections of MD have been largely conserved, though the anatomical nomenclature changes across species. Based on thalamocortical projections and cellular architecture, Ray and Price[163] identified the primate MD pars caudo-dorsalis as analogous to the rat medial and dorsolateral MD we studied.

MD has been implicated in behaviors involving integration of sensory information with affective or motivational information. These include fear conditioning,[170,171] goal directed behavior,[172] and spatial working memory tasks.[173] Most relevant to the present topic, and consistent with the notion that pain is both a sensory discriminative and an emotional experience,[19] electrophysiological studies in humans and rats indicate that MD plays an important role in processing noxious inputs.[96,148,174] These studies reveal that MD neurons are almost exclusively driven by noxious, rather than innocuous peripheral inputs.[46,96,108,174] Consistent with a role for MD in SCI-Pain, one study reports abnormal neuronal activity in MD of patients with chronic pain[148] though not much is known about properties of MD neurons in healthy humans.

These findings led to our hypothesis that pain after SCI is associated with abnormal increases in spontaneous and evoked activity of MD neurons. We recorded single and multi-unit activity from MD of either anesthetized or awake rats, and compared data from rats with SCI with data from sham-operated controls.[46] Consistent with our hypothesis, MD neurons from rats with SCI show significant increases in spontaneous firing rates; these were, on average 2.5 fold higher than those recorded from MD neurons of sham operated rats. Because MD is densely interconnected with several areas of the limbic circuit that are critical for nociceptive processing,[96,103,107,175–180] it is possible that this contributes to the ongoing spontaneous pain in this condition.

Also consistent with our hypothesis are findings that, in rats with SCI, responses in MD neurons to noxious stimuli are significantly larger in magnitude than those from sham operated rats; the magnitude of responses was nearly seven-fold higher in SCI animals than in sham-operated animals.[46] This is a larger increase than we found in the ventrobasal complex (four-fold; see above), yet smaller than that we reported for PO neurons (40 fold).

An earlier study by Dostrovsky and Guilbaud[174] examined electrophysiological activity in several midline thalamic nuclei, including MD, in anesthetized normal and arthritic rats. In agreement with our findings, they found MD neurons to respond preferentially to nociceptive stimulation, and to respond to stimulation of large, bilateral receptive fields. Though the authors' description of normal electrophysiological activity in MD agrees with what we have presented here, they found no change in spontaneous firing rate or magnitude of response in arthritic animals. The difference between their and our results is likely due to the fact that, in the arthritic model, hyperalgesia is largely driven by peripheral inflammation,[181–183] indicating that peripheral tissue damage is a driving force for maintenance of pain. In contrast, we use an animal model of SCI-Pain to produce long lasting pain characterized by a tonic aversive state, and that has significant central component.[45]

We found no difference in the proportion of MD neurons that had spontaneous burst activity (defined as described above for PO neurons) between the spinal-lesioned and sham-operated groups. Neither was there a difference in the number or frequency of bursts during spontaneous activity or of any burst property that we tested (number of action potentials per burst, inter-spike interval during burst, etc). This is consistent with our previous report on PO thalamus, where we found no change in bursting activity in animals with SCI,[45] though we and others have reported a moderate increase of bursting in first-order somatosensory nuclei (ventrobasal thalamus) in this model of SCI-Pain.[43,45] This selective change in burst activity after lesions of the STT may be a result of differential anatomical connections or physiological properties between first-order and higher-order thalamic nuclei (see Sherman and Guillery[86]).

Unexpectedly, MD neurons from both sham and spinal-lesioned animals had significantly *lower* frequency of burst firing in response to noxious peripheral stimulation, compared to spontaneous bursts. Because thalamic burst firing requires de-inactivation of T-type calcium channels, neurons only fire in burst mode when they are relatively hyperpolarized (see Sherman and Guillery[86]). It is possible that after noxious pinch, ascending excitation from the STT prevents thalamocortical neurons in MD from becoming sufficiently hyperpolarized, thereby preventing neurons from firing in burst mode in response to peripheral simulation.

Taken together, these studies demonstrate that SCI-Pain is associated not only with increased excitability of neurons in the first order, "specific" somatosensory thalamic nucleus (VP), but that even more dramatic changes occur in higher order, "associative" nuclei, the mediodorsal and posterior thalamic nuclei. Thus, chronic pain after SCI likely represents a multifaceted pathophysiology, involving converging processes in several thalamic nuclei.

As described above, there is at least one proven causal mechanism for the increased excitability of thalamic neurons after SCI—the abnormal expression of the $Na_v1.3$ channel.[92] However, the expression of this channel appears to be specific to VPL (and spinal neurons), because other thalamic nuclei were reported not to express this channel after SCI.[184] We therefore sought alternative mechanisms for the hyperexcitability we observed in PO and MD neurons.

ABNORMALITIES IN INHIBITORY INPUTS TO THALAMIC NUCLEI

More than 100 years ago, the British neurologists Sir Henry Head and Sir Gordon Holmes[55] postulated that central pain reflects "excessive response" due to processes that "free the thalamic centre from control." A modern interpretation of this postulate is that CPS—including

SCI-Pain—results from abnormally suppressed inhibition in the thalamus. However, the identity of this disinhibitory process remains unknown.[4,52]

Somatosensory thalamic nuclei in the rodent (including VP, PO and MD) contain few, if any, GABAergic interneurons.[159,185] Therefore, all GABAergic inhibition is mediated by extrinsic afferents. An important source of GABAergic afferents is the **reticular nucleus of the thalamus** (TRN) whose efferents target all three thalamic nuclei discussed here. TRN does not receive spinothalamic inputs, and its major source of excitatory input is the somatosensory cortex.[186]

A second important source of inhibitory inputs is the **zona incerta** (ZI). The ZI is aptly named: the function of this "zone of uncertainty" in the ventral thalamus has been debated since Auguste Forel first described it in 1877. ZI sends a dense GABAergic projection to both PO[126,127] and MD,[154,155] two nuclei critically involved in nociceptive processing. We have demonstrated that ZI exerts potent feed-forward and tonic inhibition of PO and MD neurons.[46,187–189] A striking feature of ZI is its target specificity: it provides inhibitory inputs *exclusively* to higher-order thalamic nuclei in the somatosensory, visual and auditory systems (e.g. PO in the somatosensory system and the pulvinar in the visual system); ZI afferents avoid first-order thalamic nuclei (e.g. VP in the somatosensory system and the lateral geniculate in the visual system).[127,154]

A third source of inhibition to the thalamus is the **anterior pretectal nucleus** (APT). Like ZI, APT exclusively innervates higher-order thalamic nuclei,[128,190] and several lines of evidence indicate that APT is involved in somatosensory functions, including nociception.[130,191–195]

Because in our model of SCI-Pain both PO and MD neuronal activity were significantly more altered than those of VP neurons (see above), we first hypothesized that the abnormally high responsiveness of PO neurons results from loss of inhibitory control from ZI.

Zona Incerta

Our findings strongly support this hypothesis. In rats with SCI-Pain, spontaneous firing of ZI neurons is 3-fold lower than normal, and responses to tactile stimuli are 50% weaker.[45] We further demonstrated that, in naïve rats, reversible inactivation of ZI results in immediate and profound hyperalgesia, and in a concomitant increased activity of MD neurons.[46] We also demonstrated that stimulation of ZI in rats with SCI results in immediate reversal of behavioral signs of hyperalgesia.[196] Thus, the suppressed spontaneous and evoked activity of ZI neurons appears to be causally related to both abnormal thalamic activity and

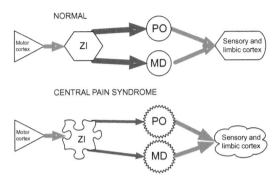

FIGURE 6.1   Schematic of the main neuronal circuit components discussed in this chapter. Green arrows represent excitatory connections, and red arrows are inhibitory. Line thickness represents the strength of the connection.

to the development of hyperalgesia in animals with SCI. Taken together with the changes described above in PO and MD of rats with SCI, these findings support the conclusion that the pathophysiology of SCI-Pain involves abnormal reduction in GABAergic inhibition of thalamic nuclei that are regulated by ZI.[18]

We concluded (see Figure 6.1) that the suppressed tonic activity of ZI neurons leads to increased spontaneous activity in PO and MD neurons, and therefore to the expression of spontaneous pain. We further concluded that the diminished evoked responses in ZI neurons results in suppressed feed-forward inhibition in PO, and therefore to hyperalgesia.

We are actively investigating the mechanisms through which SCI results in suppressed ZI activity. Preliminary findings[197] suggest that SCI is associated with a reduction of approximately 30% in the expression of GAD (the rate limiting enzyme in GABA synthesis) in ZI neurons, and a subsequent, gradual apoptosis of GABAergic neurons in ZI. Our preliminary findings also suggest that these changes result in a significant decrease in the frequency—but not the amplitude—of miniature inhibitory postsynaptic currents (mIPSCs) recorded from PO and MD neurons, supporting the conclusion that SCI results in suppression of inhibitory control of these thalamic nuclei by ZI.[197]

Anterior Pretectal Nucleus

Another source of inhibition is the anterior pretectal nucleus (APT). The APT also sends dense GABAergic inputs to higher-order thalamic nuclei and, like ZI, has been shown to regulate the activity of PO neurons.[128,130] The APT receives nociceptive inputs through the STT[198–200] and has been implicated in a variety of pain-related functions.[201,202] Indeed we found that the activity in the APT of animals with confirmed hyperalgesia after SCI is abnormal[130]: The firing rate of APT neurons is increased compared to sham-operated controls. This increase is due to a selective increase in firing of tonic neurons that project to and inhibit ZI and an increase in bursts of fast bursting and slow rhythmic neurons. These findings suggest that APT regulates ZI inputs to PO and that enhanced APT activity contributes to the hyperalgesia observed in animals after SCI.[130]

Thalamic Reticular Nucleus

We recognize that the maladapative changes we describe in ZI of SCI-Pain rats cannot directly explain the abnormal activity reported in VP thalamus of these animals. This is because ZI does not project directly to VP thalamus (see above). The predominant inhibitory input to this nucleus arises from the GABAergic reticular nucleus of the thalamus (TRN), which has been hypothesized to have a role in central pain.[203] Moreover, TRN neurons can be inhibited by noxious stimuli,[204] and the inhibitory drive from TRN upon VP neurons regulates bursting in these neurons.[205,206] Therefore, SCI-associated alterations in inhibitory inputs from TRN may also affect the activity of VP ('first order') thalamic nuclei and contribute to chronic pain.

TRN provides inhibitory inputs also to "higher order" thalamic nuclei, including PO and MD (see above). However, anatomical and electrophysiological evidence argues against a major role for TRN in mediating the maladaptive plasticity in these thalamic nuclei. TRN does not receive direct ascending sensory inputs (although it can be inhibited by noxious stimuli; see above), and its major source of excitatory input is from somatosensory cortex.[186] Further, GABAergic terminals in PO that originate from ZI differ from those of TRN origin by their larger size, the presence of multiple release sites, and multiple filamentous contacts, all features suggesting that ZI exerts significantly more potent inhibition upon PO.[128,154]

To our knowledge, the role of TRN in the pathogenesis of SCI-Pain is yet to be determined.

CORTICAL ABNORMALITIES

The perception of pain requires activity in the cerebral cortex.[104,107,207-209] Therefore, pain after SCI must involve abnormal cortical activity. However, the nature of SCI-related changes in cortical neurophysiology are relatively known. Although a few functional imaging studies have reported abnormal cortical responses in patients with central pain syndrome (CPS),[110,210-212] to our knowledge there have been no direct recordings from cortical neurons in CPS conditions. However, Jensen et al.[213] recently showed that certain EEG activity patterns may be associated with enhanced pain or with a vulnerability to experience chronic pain in persons with SCI. And Endo et al.[210,214] report that SCI-Pain is associated with increased cortical blood oxygen level dependent (BOLD) signals.

Based on our finding that PO activity is abnormally increased in CPS (see above), we expected the cortical targets of PO to show increased neuronal activity. Primary somatosensory cortex (SI) is a major projection target of PO[133,215–219] and is involved in processing sensory-discriminative aspects of nociceptive inputs.[104,220–222] We therefore tested the hypothesis that SCI is associated with increased activity in SI neurons.

Consistent with our hypothesis, SI neurons recorded from spinal lesioned rats exhibited significantly higher spontaneous firing rates and greater responses evoked by innocuous and noxious mechanical stimulation of the hindpaw, compared to control rats.[42] Neurons from lesioned rats also showed a greater tendency than controls to fire bursts of action potentials (defined as in our PO study, above) in response to noxious stimuli. Thus, the excruciatingly painful symptoms of SCI-Pain may result, at least in part, from abnormally increased activity in SI.

THALAMOCORTICAL ABNORMALITIES

As we show above, SCI-pain is associated with widespread maladaptive changes. These changes, caused by injury, deafferentation, and loss of inhibition, result in significant anatomical and neurochemical changes in cortical and subcortical structures in humans[223–225] and animals.[81,210,214,226] Thus, these changes are likely to culminate in abnormal functional interactions in brain networks involved in nociceptive processing. Therefore, we hypothesized that SCI-pain will be reflected in abnormal functional connectivity of brain areas implicated in pain processing.

To test this hypothesis, we performed a longitudinal study in a our animal model of SCI (see above) and acquired resting state functional magnetic resonance imaging (fMRI) scans, under isoflurane anesthesia, before spinal surgery and at 3, 7, 14, and 21 days after surgery in the same animals.[227] We used seed-based analysis to assess if connectivity in VPL thalamus, and SI cortex changes after SCI. This analysis revealed that functional connectivity is decreased between VPL and SI at 7 days after SCI, relative to sham-operated controls. This reduction preceded an increase in connectivity between SI and other cortical areas involved in nociceptive processing, such as the anterior cingulate cortex, insula and retrosplenial cortex (RSC). In addition, connectivity of VPL with the contralateral thalamus was increased at 7 and 14 days after SCI. The temporal pattern of increases in functional connectivity within the thalamus and between cortical areas (particularly SI and RSC) had a striking resemblance to the temporal pattern for the development of a "below-level" mechanical hyperalgesia in the same animals.[227]

These results are reminiscent of findings in patients with chronic pain, where it has been suggested that the activity of thalamic neurons is abnormally enhanced, causing them to fire synchronously at a low frequency (<5 Hz).[228] These low frequency oscillations have been shown to release neurons in the cortex from inhibition,[229] which, in turn, will cause cortical neurons to discharge in spontaneous, continuous oscillations at a higher frequency.[230]

The reduced connectivity between the thalamus and SI, and the subsequent increased connectivity between cortical areas involved in nociceptive perception suggest that SCI-pain is associated with a functional disconnection (asynchrony in brain oscillations) between the thalamus and cortex. Therefore, treatments that restore inhibition in the thalamus and re-establish normal thalamocortical rhythms may prove effective in the treatment of SCI-pain.

THERAPIES TO RESTORE INHIBITION TO THALAMIC NUCLEI

Treatment options for patients suffering from SCI-Pain have traditionally been limited to either pharmacological treatments or non pharmacologic approaches or a combination of both. A variety of medications have been used, including NSAIDS, opioids, antidepressants, anticonvulsants, NMDA receptor antagonists, alpha 2-adrenergic agonists and GABA-receptor agonists. However, these medications are rarely consistently effective, and treatment protocols that produce consistent and permanent pain relief have yet to be established.[14,231]

Non-pharmacologic approaches include electrical stimulation of various structures in the central nervous system, including the spinal cord, the internal capsule,[232] the periaqueductal gray-periventricular gray complex,[233] the somatosensory cortex and the thalamus.[234] These approaches also offer inconsistent and temporary benefits.

A potentially effective treatment for chronic neuropathic pain is electrical stimulation of the motor cortex. This method was introduced in 1991 for the treatment of central pain[235] and since then its use has been extended for the treatment of several other neuropathic pain conditions.[236–238] Motor cortex stimulation (MCS) is more effective and more advantageous than stimulating other central nervous system structures because of the low occurrence of complications[239] the lower propensity to cause seizures,[240] and because of the ability to apply it non-invasively using repetitive transcranial magnetic stimulation.[241] Pain relief occurs almost immediately after onset of motor cortex stimulation in approximately 50% of patients and persists after the stimulation has stopped.[242,243] However, mixed outcomes and varied success rates are reported.[244] The absence of well controlled studies, the diverse approaches employed, and lack of understanding of how motor cortex stimulation results in pain relief have all contributed to the mixed outcomes and reduced the enthusiasm for this potentially effective treatment.

Several hypotheses have been proposed to explain how MCS provides pain relief. Most propose that MCS enhances inhibition in one of three structures along the neural axis: (1) within the neocortex; (2) in the spinal cord; or (3) within the thalamus.[212,245,246] Advocates for a cortical mechanism of pain relief argue that MCS enhances activity of "non-nociceptive" sensory inputs in SI cortex that, in turn, inhibit nociceptive neurons in SI that receive inputs from the spinothalamic tract.[247,248] However, this notion appears at odds with results of imaging studies demonstrating that motor cortex stimulation does not cause changes in cerebral blood flow in the primary motor (MI) or somatosensory cortex.[246,249–251] There are those who argue that MCS may directly or indirectly inhibit nociceptive inputs in the spinal cord. Direct inhibition is unlikely, though, because M1 does not project to the superficial layers or to the marginal zone of the dorsal horn.[252] An indirect role is more likely, as MCS may activate descending inhibitory systems and cause endogenous opioid release.[253,254] Despite limited support for this claim, manipulations that specifically activate endogenous opioid release, such as deep brain stimulation of the periaqueductal gray, are especially poor for the treatment of central pain.[233,255] Some have hypothesized that MCS activates corticothalamic pathways, and that these, in turn, inhibit nociceptive processing in the thalamus.[256–258] In support of this hypothesis it was argued that patients responsive to GABA analogs or barbiturate treatment are more likely to benefit from motor cortex stimulation.[245,259,260] However, the specific role of the thalamus is still debated, and the source of altered inhibition, the mechanisms for engagement of inhibition, and the specific nuclei affected by MCS remain to be elucidated.

Recently, we used our animal model of SCI to study the effective parameters of motor cortex stimulation.[196] We systematically tested a large parameter space of stimulus conditions, an advantage not readily available in human studies. We found that MCS reduced hyperalgesia in a manner that is dependent on stimulation parameters and protocol used, and that stimulation at an intensity of $50\,\mu A$ and frequency of $50\,Hz$ for 30 minutes was most effective at reducing mechanical hyperalgesia in rats bilaterally.[196]

Using these effective stimulation parameters we were able to directly test mechanisms of pain relief produced by motor cortex stimulation. We discussed above evidence that activity of ZI is suppressed in conditions of SCI-Pain.[18] The ZI receives dense projections from prefrontal motor areas, including the motor cortex.[261,262] Therefore, reduction in hyperalgesia after MCS could be due to enhanced activity in ZI. To test this hypothesis, we used our animal model of SCI-pain and performed *in vivo* extracellular electrophysiological recordings from single, well-isolated neurons in anesthetized rats.[263] We recorded spontaneous activity in ZI and PO from 48 rats before, during and after MCS (50 µA, 50 Hz; 300 ms pulses). We found that MCS enhanced spontaneous activity in 35% of ZI neurons and suppressed spontaneous activity in 58% of PO neurons. The majority of MCS-enhanced ZI neurons (81%) were located in the ventrorateral subdivision of ZI—the area containing PO-projecting ZI neurons.[154,188] Inactivating ZI using muscimol (GABA$_A$ receptor agonist) blocked the effects of MCS in 73% of PO neurons.[263] In addition, we found that the administration of lidocaine, or muscimol, but not saline into ZI reversibly blocked the behavioral effects of motor cortex stimulation.[196]

These results, combined with our earlier findings[18] identify ZI as a source of inhibition that can be manipulated to produce pain relief, and describe a novel system that affects nociceptive transmission within the thalamus through corticothalamic interactions. Identifying the mechanisms involved in the short and long-term consequences of motor cortex stimulation may shift current research and clinical practice paradigms and might pave the way towards the development of molecular, pharmacologic and physiologic methods for permanent pain relief that target these structures.

Acknowledgments

Authors' work was generously supported by NINDS Research Grants R01-051799 to A.K. and R01-NS069568 to R.M., Department of Defense grant SC090126 to R.M., and the Christopher and Dana Reeve Foundation to A.K.

References

1. Persu C, Caun V, Dragomiriteanu I, Geavlete P. Urological management of the patient with traumatic spinal cord injury. *J Med Life*. 2009;2:296–302.
2. Widerstrom-Noga EG, Felix ER, Cruz-Almeida Y, Turk DC. Psychosocial subgroups in persons with spinal cord injuries and chronic pain. *Arch Phys Med Rehabil*. 2007;88:1628–1635.
3. Abramson CE, McBride KE, Konnyu KJ, Elliott SL. Sexual health outcome measures for individuals with a spinal cord injury: a systematic review. *Spinal Cord*. 2008;46:320–324.

4. Boivie J. Central pain. In: McMahon S, Koltzenburg M, eds. *Wall and Melzack's Textbook of Pain*. Oxford: Churchill Livingstone; 2005. p. 1057–1074.
5. Bowsher D. Termination of the central pain pathway in man: the conscious appreciation of pain. *Brain*. 1957;80:606–622.
6. Cruz-Almeida Y, Felix ER, Martinez-Arizala A, Widerstrom-Noga EG. Pain symptom profiles in persons with spinal cord injury. *Pain Med*. 2009;10:1246–1259.
7. Klit H, Finnerup NB, Jensen TS. Clinical characteristics of central poststroke pain. In: Henry JL, Panju A, Yashpal K, eds. *Central Neuropathic Pain: Focus on Poststroke Pain*. Seattle: IASP Press; 2007. p. 27–41.
8. Holmes G. Pain of central origin. In: Osler W, ed. *Contributions to Medical and Biological Research*. New York: Hoeber; 1919. p. 235–246.
9. Defrin R, Ohry A, Blumen N, Urca G. Pain following spinal cord injury. *Spinal Cord*. 2002;40:96–97. [author reply 98-9].
10. Stormer S, Gerner HJ, Gruninger W, et al. Chronic pain/dysaesthesiae in spinal cord injury patients: results of a multicentre study. *Spinal Cord*. 1997;35:446–455.
11. Yezierski RP. Pain following spinal cord injury: pathophysiology and central mechanisms. *Prog Brain Res*. 2000;129:429–449.
12. Greenspan JD, Ohara S, Sarlani E, Lenz FA. Allodynia in patients with post-stroke central pain (CPSP) studied by statistical quantitative sensory testing within individuals. *Pain*. 2004;109:357–366.
13. Tasker RR. Meralgia paresthetica. *J Neurosurg*. 1991;75:168.
14. Baastrup C, Finnerup NB. Pharmacological management of neuropathic pain following spinal cord injury. *CNS Drugs*. 2008;22:455–475.
15. Falci S, Best L, Bayles R, Lammertse D, Starnes C. Dorsal root entry zone microcoagulation for spinal cord injury-related central pain: operative intramedullary electrophysiological guidance and clinical outcome. *J Neurosurg*. 2002;97:193–200.
16. Rintala DH, Holmes SA, Fiess RN, Courtade D, Loubser PG. Prevalence and characteristics of chronic pain in veterans with spinal cord injury. *J Rehabil Res Dev*. 2005;42:573–584.
17. Tasker RR, DeCarvalho GT, Dolan EJ. Intractable pain of spinal cord origin: clinical features and implications for surgery. *J Neurosurg*. 1992;77:373–378.
18. Masri R, Keller A. Chronic pain following spinal cord injury. In: Jandial R, ed. *Frontiers in Spinal Cord and Spine Repair*. Austin: Landers Bioscience; 2011.
19. Merskey H, Bogduk N. *Classification of Chronic Pain: Descriptions of Chronic Pain Syndromes and Definitions of Pain Terms*. Seattle: IASP Press; 1994.
20. Bonica JJ. History of pain concepts and pain therapy. *Mt Sinai J Med*. 1991;58:191–202.
21. Lamid S, Chia JK, Kohli A, Cid E. Chronic pain in spinal cord injury: comparison between inpatients and outpatients. *Arch Phys Med Rehabil*. 1985;66:777–778.
22. Levi R, Hultling C, Nash MS, Seiger A. The Stockholm spinal cord injury study: 1. Medical problems in a regional SCI population. *Paraplegia*. 1995;33:308–315.
23. Nepomuceno C, Fine PR, Richards JS, et al. Pain in patients with spinal cord injury. *Arch Phys Med Rehabil*. 1979;60:605–609.
24. Siddall PJ, McClelland JM, Rutkowski SB, Cousins MJ. A longitudinal study of the prevalence and characteristics of pain in the first 5 years following spinal cord injury. *Pain*. 2003;103:249–257.
25. Woolsey RM. Chronic pain following spinal cord injury. *J Am Paraplegia Soc*. 1986;9:39–41.
26. Levitt M, Levitt JH. The deafferentation syndrome in monkeys: dysesthesias of spinal origin. *Pain*. 1981;10:129–147.
27. Vierck CJJ, Greenspan JD, Ritz LA. Long-term changes in purposive and reflexive responses to nociceptive stimulation following anterolateral chordotomy. *J Neurosci*. 1990;10:2077–2095.

28. Vierck CJJ, Light AR. Effects of combined hemotoxic and anterolateral spinal lesions on nociceptive sensitivity. *Pain*. 1999;83:447–457.

29. Beattie MS, Bresnahan JC, Komon J, et al. Endogenous repair after spinal cord contusion injuries in the rat. *Exp Neurol*. 1997;148:453–463.

30. Hulsebosch CE, Hains BC, Crown ED, Carlton SM. Mechanisms of chronic central neuropathic pain after spinal cord injury. *Brain Res Rev*. 2009;60:202–213.

31. Sharp K, Boroujerdi A, Steward O, Luo ZD. A rat chronic pain model of spinal cord contusion injury. *Methods Mol Biol*. 2012;851:195–203.

32. Scheff SW, Rabchevsky AG, Fugaccia I, Main JA, Lumpp JEJ. Experimental modeling of spinal cord injury: characterization of a force-defined injury device. *J Neurotrauma*. 2003;20:179–193.

33. Yoon YW, Dong H, Arends JJ, Jacquin MF. Mechanical and cold allodynia in a rat spinal cord contusion model. *Somatosens Mot Res*. 2004;21:25–31.

34. Christensen MD, Everhart AW, Pickelman JT, Hulsebosch CE. Mechanical and thermal allodynia in chronic central pain following spinal cord injury. *Pain*. 1996;68:97–107.

35. Christensen MD, Hulsebosch CE. Chronic central pain after spinal cord injury. *J Neurotrauma*. 1997;14:517–537.

36. Caudle RM, Perez FM, King C, Yu CG, Yezierski RP. N-methyl-D-aspartate receptor subunit expression and phosphorylation following excitotoxic spinal cord injury in rats. *Neurosci Lett*. 2003;349:37–40.

37. Yezierski RP, Liu S, Ruenes GL, Kajander KJ, Brewer KL. Excitotoxic spinal cord injury: behavioral and morphological characteristics of a central pain model. *Pain*. 1998;75:141–155.

38. Hao JX, Xu XJ. Treatment of a chronic allodynia-like response in spinally injured rats: effects of systemically administered excitatory amino acid receptor antagonists. *Pain*. 1996;66:279–285.

39. Hao JX, Xu XJ, Yu YX, Seiger A, Wiesenfeld-Hallin Z. Hypersensitivity of dorsal horn wide dynamic range neurons to cutaneous mechanical stimuli after transient spinal cord ischemia in the rat. *Neurosci Lett*. 1991;128:105–108.

40. Wieseler J, Ellis A, Sprunger D, et al. A novel method for modeling facial allodynia associated with migraine in awake and freely moving rats. *J Neurosci Methods*. 2010;185:236–245.

41. Moore CI, Cao R. The hemo-neural hypothesis: on the role of blood flow in information processing. *J Neurophysiol*. 2008;99:2035–2047.

42. Quiton RL, Masri R, Thompson SM, Keller A. Abnormal activity of primary somatosensory cortex in central pain syndrome. *J Neurophysiol*. 2010;104:1717–1725.

43. Wang G, Thompson SM. Maladaptive homeostatic plasticity in a rodent model of central pain syndrome: thalamic hyperexcitability after spinothalamic tract lesions. *J Neurosci*. 2008;28:11959–11969.

44. Finnerup NB, Johannesen IL, Sindrup SH, Bach FW, Jensen TS. Pain and dysesthesia in patients with spinal cord injury: a postal survey. *Spinal Cord*. 2001;39:256–262.

45. Masri R, Quiton RL, Lucas JM, Murray PD, Thompson SM, Keller A. Zona incerta: a role in central pain. *J Neurophysiol*. 2009;102:181–191.

46. Whitt JL, Masri R, Pulimood NS, Keller A. Pathological activity in mediodorsal thalamus of rats with spinal cord injury pain. *J Neurosci*. 2013;33:3915–3926.

47. Mogil JS. Animal models of pain: progress and challenges. *Nat Rev Neurosci*. 2009;10:283–294.

48. King T, Vera-Portocarrero L, Gutierrez T, et al. Unmasking the tonic-aversive state in neuropathic pain. *Nat Neurosci*. 2009;12:1364–1366.

49. Davoody L, Quiton RL, Lucas JM, Ji Y, Keller A, Masri R. Conditioned place preference reveals tonic pain in an animal model of central pain. *J Pain*. 2011;12:868–874.

50. Edinger L. Giebt es central entstehende Schmerzen? *Deutsche Zeitschrift für Nervenheilkunde.* 1891;1:262–282.
51. Greiff F. Zur Localisation der Hemichorea. *Arch Psychol Nervenkr.* 1883;14:598–624.
52. Canavero S, Bonicalzi V. *Central Pain Syndrome: Pathophysiology, Diagnosis and Management.* New York: Cambridge Univ Press; 2007.
53. Fregni F, Freedman S, Pascual-Leone A. Recent advances in the treatment of chronic pain with non-invasive brain stimulation techniques. *Lancet Neurol.* 2007;6:188–191.
54. Dejerine J, Roussy G. Le syndrome thalamique. *Rev Neurol.* 1906;15:521–532.
55. Head H, Holmes G. Sensory disturbances from cerebral lesions. *Brain.* 1911;34:102–254.
56. Bowsher D. Central pain. *Pain Rev.* 1995;2:175–186.
57. Finnerup NB, Johannesen IL, Bach FW, Jensen TS. Sensory function above lesion level in spinal cord injury patients with and without pain. *Somatosens Mot Res.* 2003;20:71–76.
58. Kim JH, Greenspan JD, Coghill RC, Ohara S, Lenz FA. Lesions limited to the human thalamic principal somatosensory nucleus (ventral caudal) are associated with loss of cold sensations and central pain. *J Neurosci.* 2007;27:4995–5004.
59. MacGowan DJ, Janal MN, Clark WC, et al. Central poststroke pain and Wallenberg's lateral medullary infarction: frequency, character, and determinants in 63 patients. *Neurology.* 1997;49:120–125.
60. Schmahmann JD, Leifer D. Parietal pseudothalamic pain syndrome. Clinical features and anatomic correlates. *Arch Neurol.* 1992;49:1032–1037.
61. Jones EG. *The Thalamus.* Cambridge: Cambridge Univ. Press; 2007.
62. Cruz-Almeida Y, Felix ER, Martinez-Arizala A, Widerstrom-Noga EG. Decreased spinothalamic and dorsal column medial lemniscus-mediated function is associated with neuropathic pain after spinal cord injury. *J Neurotrauma.* 2012;29:2706–2715.
63. Beric A. Post-spinal cord injury pain states. *Pain.* 1997;72:295–298.
64. Finnerup NB. A review of central neuropathic pain states. *Curr Opin Anaesthesiol.* 2008;21:586–589.
65. Finnerup NB, Jensen TS. Spinal cord injury pain—mechanisms and treatment. *Eur J Neurol.* 2004;11:73–82.
66. Gwak YS, Hulsebosch CE. Neuronal hyperexcitability: a substrate for central neuropathic pain after spinal cord injury. *Curr Pain Headache Rep.* 2011;15:215–222.
67. Vierck CJJ, Siddall P, Yezierski RP. Pain following spinal cord injury: animal models and mechanistic studies. *Pain.* 2000;89:1–5.
68. Wu J, Stoica BA, Faden AI. Cell cycle activation and spinal cord injury. *Neurotherapeutics.* 2011;8:221–228.
69. Yezierski RP. Spinal cord injury pain: spinal and supraspinal mechanisms. *JRRD.* 2009;46:95.
70. Zhao P, Waxman SG, Hains BC. Modulation of thalamic nociceptive processing after spinal cord injury through remote activation of thalamic microglia by cysteine cysteine chemokine ligand 21. *J Neurosci.* 2007;27:8893–8902.
71. Porreca F, Ossipov MH, Gebhart GF. Chronic pain and medullary descending facilitation. *Trends Neurosci.* 2002;25:319–325.
72. Denkers MR, Biagi HL, Ann OBM, Jadad AR, Gauld ME. Dorsal root entry zone lesioning used to treat central neuropathic pain in patients with traumatic spinal cord injury: a systematic review. *Spine (Phila Pa 1976).* 2002;27:E177–E184.
73. Que JC, Siddall PJ, Cousins MJ. Pain management in a patient with intractable spinal cord injury pain: a case report and literature review. *Anesth Analg.* 2007;105:1462–1473.
74. Lenz FA, Kwan HC, Dostrovsky JO, Tasker RR. Characteristics of the bursting pattern of action potentials that occurs in the thalamus of patients with central pain. *Brain Res.* 1989;496:357–360.
75. Lenz FA, Tasker RR, Dostrovsky JO, et al. Abnormal single-unit activity recorded in the somatosensory thalamus of a quadriplegic patient with central pain. *Pain.* 1987;31:225–236.

76. Foerster O. *Die Lactungsbahnen des Schmerzgefuhls und die chirurgische Behandlung der Schmerzzustande*. Berlin: Urban and Schwarzenberg; 1927.

77. Craig AD. Mechanisms of thalamic pain. In: Henry JL, Panju A, Yashpal K, eds. *Central Neuropathic Pain: Focus on Poststroke Pain*. Seattle: IASP Press; 2007. p. 81–99.

78. Apkarian AV, Shi T, Bruggemann J, Airapetian LR. Segregation of nociceptive and non-nociceptive networks in the squirrel monkey somatosensory thalamus. *J Neurophysiol*. 2000;84:484–494.

79. Zhang X, Davidson S, Giesler GJJ. Thermally identified subgroups of marginal zone neurons project to distinct regions of the ventral posterior lateral nucleus in rats. *J Neurosci*. 2006;26:5215–5223.

80. Graziano A, Jones EG. Widespread thalamic terminations of fibers arising in the superficial medullary dorsal horn of monkeys and their relation to calbindin immunoreactivity. *J Neurosci*. 2004;24:248–256.

81. Anderson WS, O'Hara S, Lawson HC, Treede RD, Lenz FA. Plasticity of pain-related neuronal activity in the human thalamus. *Prog Brain Res*. 2006;157:353–364.

82. Pattany PM, Yezierski RP, Widerstrom-Noga EG, et al. Proton magnetic resonance spectroscopy of the thalamus in patients with chronic neuropathic pain after spinal cord injury. *AJNR Am J Neuroradiol*. 2002;23:901–905.

83. Weng HR, Lee JI, Lenz FA, et al. Functional plasticity in primate somatosensory thalamus following chronic lesion of the ventral lateral spinal cord. *Neuroscience*. 2000;101:393–401.

84. Hains BC, Saab CY, Waxman SG. Changes in electrophysiological properties and sodium channel Nav1.3 expression in thalamic neurons after spinal cord injury. *Brain*. 2005;128:2359–2371.

85. Hubscher CH, Johnson RD. Chronic spinal cord injury induced changes in the responses of thalamic neurons. *Exp Neurol*. 2006;197:177–188.

86. Sherman SM, Guillery RW. *Exploring the Thalamus and its Role in Cortical Function*. Cambridge: MIT Press; 2005.

87. Apkarian AV, Shi T. Squirrel monkey lateral thalamus. I. Somatic nociresponsive neurons and their relation to spinothalamic terminals. *J Neurosci*. 1994;14:6779–6795.

88. Berkley KJ. Specific somatic sensory relays in the mammalian diencephalon. *Rev Neurol (Paris)*. 1986;142:283–290.

89. Price DD. Central neural mechanisms that interrelate sensory and affective dimensions of pain. *Mol Interv*. 2002;2:392–403.

90. Dib-Hajj SD, Cummins TR, Black JA, Waxman SG. Sodium channels in normal and pathological pain. *Annu Rev Neurosci*. 2010;33:325–347.

91. Hains BC, Saab CY, Waxman SG. Alterations in burst firing of thalamic VPL neurons and reversal by Na(v)1.3 antisense after spinal cord injury. *J Neurophysiol*. 2006;95:3343–3352.

92. Hains BC, Waxman SG. Sodium channel expression and the molecular pathophysiology of pain after SCI. *Prog Brain Res*. 2007;161:195–203.

93. Iwata M, LeBlanc BW, Kadasi LM, Zerah ML, Cosgrove RG, Saab CY. High-frequency stimulation in the ventral posterolateral thalamus reverses electrophysiologic changes and hyperalgesia in a rat model of peripheral neuropathic pain. *Pain*. 2011;152:2505–2513.

94. Gerke MB, Duggan AW, Xu L, Siddall PJ. Thalamic neuronal activity in rats with mechanical allodynia following contusive spinal cord injury. *Neuroscience*. 2003;117:715–722.

95. Lee JI, Ohara S, Dougherty PM, Lenz FA. Pain and temperature encoding in the human thalamic somatic sensory nucleus (Ventral caudal): inhibition-related bursting evoked by somatic stimuli. *J Neurophysiol*. 2005;94:1676–1687.

96. Wang JY, Luo F, Chang JY, Woodward DJ, Han JS. Parallel pain processing in freely moving rats revealed by distributed neuron recording. *Brain Res*. 2003;992:263–271.

97. Dostrovsky JO. The thalamus and human pain. In: Henry JL, Panju A, Yashpal K, eds. *Central Neuropathic Pain: Focus on Poststroke Pain.* Seattle: IASP Press; 2007. p. 101–112.

98. Gorecki J, Hirayama T, Dostrovsky JO, Tasker RR, Lenz FA. Thalamic stimulation and recording in patients with deafferentation and central pain. *Stereotact Funct Neurosurg.* 1989;52:219–226.

99. Hirayama T, Dostrovsky JO, Gorecki J, Tasker RR, Lenz FA. Recordings of abnormal activity in patients with deafferentation and central pain. *Stereotact Funct Neurosurg.* 1989;52:120–126.

100. Jahnsen H, Llinas R. Electrophysiological properties of guinea-pig thalamic neurones: an in vitro study. *J Physiol.* 1984;349:205–226.

101. Melzack R, Casey KL. Sensory, motivational and central control determinants of pain. In: Kenshalo DR, ed. *The Skin Senses.* Springfield: Thomas; 1968. p. 423–439.

102. Price DD. *Psychological Mechanisms of Pain and Analgesia.* Seattle: I.A.S.P. Press; 1999.

103. Treede RD, Kenshalo DR, Gracely RH, Jones AK. The cortical representation of pain. *Pain.* 1999;79:105–111.

104. Apkarian AV, Bushnell MC, Treede RD, Zubieta JK. Human brain mechanisms of pain perception and regulation in health and disease. *Eur J Pain.* 2005;9:463–484.

105. Melzack R. From the gate to the neuromatrix. *Pain.* 1999(suppl 6):S121–S126.

106. Hodge CJJ, Apkarian AV. The spinothalamic tract. *Crit Rev Neurobiol.* 1990;5:363–397.

107. Treede RD, Apkarian AV, Bromm B, Greenspan JD, Lenz FA. Cortical representation of pain: functional characterization of nociceptive areas near the lateral sulcus. *Pain.* 2000;87:113–119.

108. Bushnell MC, Duncan GH. Sensory and affective aspects of pain perception: is medial thalamus restricted to emotional issues?. *Exp Brain Res.* 1989;78:415–418.

109. Baliki MN, Geha PY, Apkarian AV. Spontaneous pain and brain activity in neuropathic pain: functional MRI and pharmacologic functional MRI studies. *Curr Pain Headache Rep.* 2007;11:171–177.

110. Ducreux D, Attal N, Parker F, Bouhassira D. Mechanisms of central neuropathic pain: a combined psychophysical and fMRI study in syringomyelia. *Brain.* 2006;129:963–976.

111. Lorenz J, Minoshima S, Casey KL. Keeping pain out of mind: the role of the dorsolateral prefrontal cortex in pain modulation. *Brain.* 2003;126:1079–1091.

112. Cusick C. Thalamic systems and the diversity of cortical areas. In: Schüz A, Miller R, eds. *Cortical Areas: Unity and Diversity.* London: Harwood Academic; 2002. p. 155–178.

113. Erickson RP, Hall WC, Jane JA, Snyder M, Diamond IT. Organization of the posterior dorsal thalamus of the hedgehog. *J Comp Neurol.* 1967;131:103–130.

114. Fukushima T, Kerr FW. Organization of trigeminothalamic tracts and other thalamic afferent systems of the brainstem in the rat: presence of gelatinosa neurons with thalamic connections. *J Comp Neurol.* 1979;183:169–184.

115. Gauriau C, Bernard JF. Posterior triangular thalamic neurons convey nociceptive messages to the secondary somatosensory and insular cortices in the rat. *J Neurosci.* 2004;24:752–761.

116. Kemplay S, Webster KE. A quantitative study of the projections of the gracile, cuneate and trigeminal nuclei and of the medullary reticular formation to the thalamus in the rat. *Neuroscience.* 1989;32:153–167.

117. Lund RD, Webster KE. Thalamic afferents from the spinal cord and trigeminal nuclei. An experimental anatomical study in the rat. *J Comp Neurol.* 1967;130:313–328.

118. Peschanski M, Ralston III HJ. Light and electron microscopic evidence of transneuronal labeling with WGA-HRP to trace somatosensory pathways to the thalamus. *J Comp Neuro.* 1985;236:29–41.

119. Peschanski M, Roudier F, Ralston III HJ, Besson JM. Ultrastructural analysis of the terminals of various somatosensory pathways in the ventrobasal complex of the rat

thalamus: an electron- microscopic study using wheatgerm agglutinin conjugated to horseradish peroxidase as an axonal tracer. *Somatosens Res.* 1985;3:75–87.

120. Ring G, Ganchrow D. Projections of nucleus caudalis and spinal cord to brainstem and diencephalon in the hedgehog (Erinaceus europaeus and Paraechinus aethiopicus): a degeneration study. *J Comp Neurol.* 1983;216:132–151.

121. Rockel AJ, Heath CJ, Jones EG. Afferent connections to the diencephalon in the marsupial phalanger and question of sensory convergence in the "posterior group" of the thalamus. *J Comp Neurol.* 1972;145:105–129.

122. Dado RJ, Giesler GJJ. Afferent input to nucleus submedius in rats: retrograde labeling of neurons in the spinal cord and caudal medulla. *J Neurosci.* 1990;10:2672–2686.

123. Iwata K, Kenshalo DRJ, Dubner R, Nahin RL. Diencephalic projections from the superficial and deep laminae of the medullary dorsal horn in the rat. *J Comp Neurol.* 1992;321:404–420.

124. Ledoux JE, Ruggiero DA, Forest R, Stornetta R, Reis DJ. Topographic organization of convergent projections to the thalamus from the inferior colliculus and spinal cord in the rat. *J Comp Neurol.* 1987;264:123–146.

125. Roger M, Cadusseau J. Afferent connections of the nucleus posterior thalami in the rat, with some evolutionary and functional considerations. *J Hirnforsch.* 1984;25:473–485.

126. Bartho P, Slezia A, Varga V, et al. Cortical control of zona incerta. *J Neurosci.* 2007;27:1670–1681.

127. Power BD, Kolmac CI, Mitrofanis J. Evidence for a large projection from the zona incerta to the dorsal thalamus. *J Comp Neurol.* 1999;404:554–565.

128. Bokor H, Frere SG, Eyre MD, et al. Selective GABAergic control of higher-order thalamic relays. *Neuron.* 2005;45:929–940.

129. Giber K, Slezia A, Bokor H, et al. Heterogeneous output pathways link the anterior pretectal nucleus with the zona incerta and the thalamus in rat. *J Comp Neurol.* 2008;506:122–140.

130. Murray PD, Masri R, Keller A. Abnormal anterior pretectal nucleus activity contributes to central pain syndrome. *J Neurophysiol.* 2010;103:3044–3053.

131. Bourassa J, Pinault D, Deschenes M. Corticothalamic projections from the cortical barrel field to the somatosensory thalamus in rats: a single-fibre study using biocytin as an anterograde tracer. *Eur J Neurosci.* 1995;7:19–30.

132. Carvell GE, Simons DJ. Thalamic and corticocortical connections of the second somatic sensory area of the mouse. *J Comp Neurol.* 1987;265:409–427.

133. Fabri M, Burton H. Topography of connections between primary somatosensory cortex and posterior complex in rat: a multiple fluorescent tracer study. *Brain Res.* 1991;538:351–357.

134. Spreafico R, Barbaresi P, Weinberg RJ, Rustioni A. SII-projecting neurons in the rat thalamus: a single- and double-retrograde-tracing study. *Somatosens Res.* 1987;4:359–375.

135. Wise SP, Jones EG. Cells of origin and terminal distribution of descending projections of the rat somatic sensory cortex. *J Comp Neurol.* 1977;175:129–157.

136. Linke R, Braune G, Schwegler H. Differential projection of the posterior paralaminar thalamic nuclei to the amygdaloid complex in the rat. *Exp Brain Res.* 2000;134:520–532.

137. Poggio GF, Mountcastle VB. A study of the functional contributions of the lemniscal and spinothalamic systems to somatic sensibility. Central nervous mechanisms in pain. *Bull Johns Hopkins Hosp.* 1960;106:266–316.

138. Berkley KJ. Response properties of cells in ventrobasal and posterior group nuclei of the cat. *J Neurophysiol.* 1973;36:940–952.

139. Calma I. Thalamo-cortical relations in the sensory nuclei of the cat. *Nature.* 1965;205:394–396.

140. Casey KL. Unit analysis of nociceptive mechanisms in the thalamus of the awake squirrel monkey. *J Neurophysiol*. 1966;29:727–750.

141. Curry MJ. The exteroceptive properties of neurones in the somatic part of the posterior group (PO). *Brain Res*. 1972;44:439–462.

142. Curry MJ, Gordon G. The spinal input to the posterior group in the cat. An electrophysiological investigation. *Brain Res*. 1972;44:427–437.

143. Perl ER, Whitlock DG. Somatic stimuli exciting spinothalamic projections to thalamic neurons in cat and monkey. *Exp Neurol*. 1961;3:256–296.

144. Rowe MJ, Sessle BJ. Somatic afferent input to posterior thalamic neurones and their axon projection to the cerebral cortex in the cat. *J Physiol*. 1968;196:19–35.

145. Whitlock DG, Perl ER. Thalamic projections of spinothalamic pathways in monkey. *Exp Neurol*. 1961;3:240–255.

146. Sherman SM. The thalamus is more than just a relay. *Curr Opin Neurobiol*. 2007;17:417–422.

147. Guido W, Lu SM, Vaughan JW, Godwin DW, Sherman SM. Receiver operating characteristic (ROC) analysis of neurons in the cat's lateral geniculate nucleus during tonic and burst response mode. *Vis Neurosci*. 1995;12:723–741.

148. Rinaldi PC, Young RF, Albe-Fessard D, Chodakiewitz J. Spontaneous neuronal hyperactivity in the medial and intralaminar thalamic nuclei of patients with deafferentation pain. *J Neurosurg*. 1991;74:415–421.

149. Sherman SM. Dual response modes in lateral geniculate neurons: mechanisms and functions. *Vis Neurosci*. 1996;13:205–213.

150. Craig AD, Kniffki KD. Spinothalamic lumbosacral lamina I cells responsive to skin and muscle stimulation in the cat. *J Physiol*. 1985;365:197–221.

151. Craig ADJ, Burton H. Spinal and medullary lamina I projection to nucleus submedius in medial thalamus: a possible pain center. *J Neurophysiol*. 1981;45:443–466.

152. Mantyh PW. The terminations of the spinothalamic tract in the cat. *Neurosci Lett*. 1983;38:119–124.

153. Peschanski M, Guilbaud G, Gautron M. Posterior intralaminar region in rat: neuronal responses to noxious and nonnoxious cutaneous stimuli. *Exp Neurol*. 1981;72:226–238.

154. Bartho P, Freund TF, Acsady L. Selective GABAergic innervation of thalamic nuclei from zona incerta. *Eur J Neurosci*. 2002;16:999–1014.

155. Erickson SL, Melchitzky DS, Lewis DA. Subcortical afferents to the lateral mediodorsal thalamus in cynomolgus monkeys. *Neuroscience*. 2004;129:675–690.

156. Aggleton JP, Mishkin M. Projections of the amygdala to the thalamus in the cynomolgus monkey. *J Comp Neurol*. 1984;222:56–68.

157. Krettek JE, Price JL. Projections from the amygdaloid complex to the cerebral cortex and thalamus in the rat and cat. *J Comp Neurol*. 1977;172:687–722.

158. Krettek JE, Price JL. The cortical projections of the mediodorsal nucleus and adjacent thalamic nuclei in the rat. *J Comp Neurol*. 1977;171:157–191.

159. Kuroda M, Lopez-Mascaraque L, Price JL. Neuronal and synaptic composition of the mediodorsal thalamic nucleus in the rat: a light and electron microscopic Golgi study. *J Comp Neurol*. 1992;326:61–81.

160. Kuroda M, Price JL. Synaptic organization of projections from basal forebrain structures to the mediodorsal thalamic nucleus of the rat. *J Comp Neurol*. 1991;303:513–533.

161. Nauta WJ. Fibre degeneration following lesions of the amygdaloid complex in the monkey. *J Anat*. 1961;95:515–531.

162. Porrino LJ, Crane AM, Goldman-Rakic PS. Direct and indirect pathways from the amygdala to the frontal lobe in rhesus monkeys. *J Comp Neurol*. 1981;198:121–136.

163. Ray JP, Price JL. The organization of projections from the mediodorsal nucleus of the thalamus to orbital and medial prefrontal cortex in macaque monkeys. *J Comp Neurol*. 1993;337:1–31.

164. Russchen FT, Amaral DG, Price JL. The afferent input to the magnocellular division of the mediodorsal thalamic nucleus in the monkey, Macaca fascicularis. *J Comp Neurol.* 1987;256:175–210.

165. Jackson JC, Benjamin RM. Unit discharges in the mediodorsal nucleus of the rabbit evoked by electrical stimulation of the olfactory bulb. *Brain Res.* 1974;75:193–201.

166. Price JL, Slotnick BM. Dual olfactory representation in the rat thalamus: an anatomical and electrophysiological study. *J Comp Neurol.* 1983;215:63–77.

167. Ilinsky IA, Jouandet ML, Goldman-Rakic PS. Organization of the nigrothalamocortical system in the rhesus monkey. *J Comp Neurol.* 1985;236:315–330.

168. Benevento LA, Fallon JH. The ascending projections of the superior colliculus in the rhesus monkey (Macaca mulatta). *J Comp Neurol.* 1975;160:339–361.

169. Risold PY, Thompson RH, Swanson LW. The structural organization of connections between hypothalamus and cerebral cortex. *Brain Res Brain Res Rev.* 1997;24:197–254.

170. Garcia R, Chang CH, Maren S. Electrolytic lesions of the medial prefrontal cortex do not interfere with long-term memory of extinction of conditioned fear. *Learn Mem.* 2006;13:14–17.

171. Li XB, Inoue T, Nakagawa S, Koyama T. Effect of mediodorsal thalamic nucleus lesion on contextual fear conditioning in rats. *Brain Res.* 2004;1008:261–272.

172. Ostlund SB, Balleine BW. Differential involvement of the basolateral amygdala and mediodorsal thalamus in instrumental action selection. *J Neurosci.* 2008;28:4398–4405.

173. Bailey KR, Mair RG. Lesions of specific and nonspecific thalamic nuclei affect prefrontal cortex-dependent aspects of spatial working memory. *Behav Neurosci.* 2005;119:410–419.

174. Dostrovsky JO, Guilbaud G. Nociceptive responses in medial thalamus of the normal and arthritic rat. *Pain.* 1990;40:93–104.

175. Jasmin L, Burkey AR, Granato A, Ohara PT. Rostral agranular insular cortex and pain areas of the central nervous system: a tract-tracing study in the rat. *J Comp Neurol.* 2004;468:425–440.

176. Johansen JP, Fields HL, Manning BH. The affective component of pain in rodents: direct evidence for a contribution of the anterior cingulate cortex. *Proc Natl Acad Sci USA.* 2001;98:8077–8082.

177. Price DD. Psychological and neural mechanisms of the affective dimension of pain. *Science.* 2000;288:1769–1772.

178. Shyu BC, Vogt BA. Short-term synaptic plasticity in the nociceptive thalamic-anterior cingulate pathway. *Mol Pain.* 2009;5:51.

179. Wang JY, Zhang HT, Han JS, Chang JY, Woodward DJ, Luo F. Differential modulation of nociceptive neural responses in medial and lateral pain pathways by peripheral electrical stimulation: a multichannel recording study. *Brain Res.* 2004;1014:197–208.

180. Zhang Y, Wang N, Wang JY, Chang JY, Woodward DJ, Luo F. Ensemble encoding of nociceptive stimulus intensity in the rat medial and lateral pain systems. *Mol Pain.* 2011;7:64.

181. Capetola RJ, Shriver DA, Rosenthale ME. Suprofen, a new peripheral analgesic. *J Pharmacol Exp Ther.* 1980;214:16–23.

182. Hirose K, Jyoyama H. Measurement of arthritic pain and effects of analgesics in the adjuvant-treated rat. *Jpn J Pharmacol.* 1971;21:717–720.

183. Winter CA, Kling PJ, Tocco DJ, Tanabe K. Analgesic activity of diflunisal [MK-647; 5-(2,4-difluorophenyl)salicylic acid] in rats with hyperalgesia induced by Freund's adjuvant. *J Pharmacol Exp Ther.* 1979;211:678–685.

184. Zhao P, Waxman SG, Hains BC. Sodium channel expression in the ventral posterolateral nucleus of the thalamus after peripheral nerve injury. *Mol Pain.* 2006;2:27.

185. Barbaresi P, Spreafico R, Frassoni C, Rustioni A. GABAergic neurons are present in the dorsal column nuclei but not in the ventroposterior complex of rats. *Brain Res.* 1986;382:305–326.

186. Liu XB, Jones EG. Predominance of corticothalamic synaptic inputs to thalamic reticular nucleus neurons in the rat. *J Comp Neurol*. 1999;414:67–79.
187. Masri R, Trageser JC, Bezdudnaya T, Li Y, Keller A. Cholinergic regulation of the posterior medial thalamic nucleus. *J Neurophysiol*. 2006;96:2265–2273.
188. Trageser JC, Burke KA, Masri R, Li Y, Sellers L, Keller A. State-dependent gating of sensory inputs by zona incerta. *J Neurophysiol*. 2006;96:1456–1463.
189. Trageser JC, Keller A. Reducing the uncertainty: gating of peripheral inputs by zona incerta. *J Neurosci*. 2004;24:8911–8915.
190. Wanaverbecq N, Bodor AL, Bokor H, Slezia A, Luthi A, Acsady L. Contrasting the functional properties of GABAergic axon terminals with single and multiple synapses in the thalamus. *J Neurosci*. 2008;28:11848–11861.
191. Berkley KJ, Mash DC. Somatic sensory projections to the pretectum in the cat. *Brain Res*. 1978;158:445–449.
192. Brandao ML, Rees H, Witt S, Roberts MH. Central antiaversive and antinociceptive effects of anterior pretectal nucleus stimulation: attenuation of autonomic and aversive effects of medial hypothalamic stimulation. *Brain Res*. 1991;542:266–272.
193. Prado WA, Faganello FA. The anterior pretectal nucleus participates as a relay station in the glutamate-, but not morphine-induced antinociception from the dorsal raphe nucleus in rats. *Pain*. 2000;88:169–176.
194. Rees H, Roberts MH. The anterior pretectal nucleus: a proposed role in sensory processing. *Pain*. 1993;53:121–135.
195. Villarreal CF, Prado WA. Modulation of persistent nociceptive inputs in the anterior pretectal nucleus of the rat. *Pain*. 2007;132:42–52.
196. Lucas JM, Ji Y, Masri R. Motor cortex stimulation reduces hyperalgesia in an animal model of central pain. *Pain*. 2011;152:1398–1407.
197. Keller A, Thalamic and cortical plasticity in pain models. Neuroscience Meeting Planner, Program No. 524.05. Online. 2011.
198. Apkarian AV, Hodge CJ. Primate spinothalamic pathways: III. Thalamic terminations of the dorsolateral and ventral spinothalamic pathways. *J Comp Neurol*. 1989;288:493–511.
199. Craig AD. Distribution of trigeminothalamic and spinothalamic lamina I terminations in the macaque monkey. *J Comp Neurol*. 2004;477:119–148.
200. Shaw VE, Mitrofanis J. Lamination of spinal cells projecting to the zona incerta of rats. *J Neurocytol*. 2001;30:695–704.
201. Porro CA, Cavazzuti M, Lui F, Giuliani D, Pellegrini M, Baraldi P. Independent time courses of supraspinal nociceptive activity and spinally mediated behavior during tonic pain. *Pain*. 2003;104:291–301.
202. Yen CT, Fu TC, Chen RC. Distribution of thalamic nociceptive neurons activated from the tail of the rat. *Brain Res*. 1989;498:118–122.
203. Foix C, Thevenard A, Nicolesco M. Algie faciale d'origine bulbo-trigéminale au cours de la syringomyélie. Troubles sympathiques concomitants. Douleur á type cellulaire. *Rev Neurol*. 1922;29:990–999.
204. Yen CT, Shaw FZ. Reticular thalamic responses to nociceptive inputs in anesthetized rats. *Brain Res*. 2003;968:179–191.
205. Halassa MM, Siegle JH, Ritt JT, Ting JT, Feng G, Moore CI. Selective optical drive of thalamic reticular nucleus generates thalamic bursts and cortical spindles. *Nat Neurosci*. 2011;14:1118–1120.
206. Steriade M. Corticothalamic resonance, states of vigilance and mentation. *Neuroscience*. 2000;101:243–276.
207. Kenshalo DR, Willis WD. The role of the cerebral cortex in pain sensation. Normal and altered states of function. *Cereb Cortex*. 1991;9:153–212.
208. Seminowicz DA, Laferriere AL, Millecamps M, Yu JS, Coderre TJ, Bushnell MC. MRI structural brain changes associated with sensory and emotional function in a rat model of long-term neuropathic pain. *Neuroimage*. 2009;47:1007–1014.

209. Vierck CJ, Whitsel BL, Favorov OV, Brown AW, Tommerdahl M. Role of primary somatosensory cortex in the coding of pain. *Pain*. 2012 [in press].

210. Endo T, Spenger C, Hao J, et al. Functional MRI of the brain detects neuropathic pain in experimental spinal cord injury. *Pain*. 2008;138:292–300.

211. Hirato M, Horikoshi S, Kawashima Y, Satake K, Shibasaki T, Ohye C. The possible role of the cerebral cortex adjacent to the central sulcus for the genesis of central (thalamic) pain--a metabolic study. *Acta Neurochir Suppl (Wien)*. 1993;58:141–144.

212. Peyron R, Laurent B, Garcia-Larrea L. Functional imaging of brain responses to pain. A review and meta-analysis (2000). *Neurophysiol Clin*. 2000;30:263–288.

213. Jensen MP, Sherlin LH, Gertz KJ, et al. Brain EEG activity correlates of chronic pain in persons with spinal cord injury: clinical implications. *Spinal Cord*. 2012

214. Endo T, Spenger C, Tominaga T, Brene S, Olson L. Cortical sensory map rearrangement after spinal cord injury: fMRI responses linked to Nogo signalling. *Brain*. 2007;130:2951–2961.

215. Bureau I, von Saint Paul F, Svoboda K. Interdigitated paralemniscal and lemniscal pathways in the mouse barrel cortex. *PLoS Biol*. 2006;4:e382.

216. Chmielowska J, Carvell GE, Simons DJ. Spatial organization of thalamocortical and corticothalamic projection systems in the rat SmI barrel cortex. *J Comp Neurol*. 1989;285:325–338.

217. Koralek KA, Jensen KF, Killackey HP. Evidence for two complementary patterns of thalamic input to the rat somatosensory cortex. *Brain Res*. 1988;463:346–351.

218. Lu SM, Lin RC. Thalamic afferents of the rat barrel cortex: a light- and electron-microscopic study using Phaseolus vulgaris leucoagglutinin as an anterograde tracer. *Somatosens Mot Res*. 1993;10:1–16.

219. Nothias F, Peschanski M, Besson JM. Somatotopic reciprocal connections between the somatosensory cortex and the thalamic Po nucleus in the rat. *Brain Res*. 1988;447:169–174.

220. Bushnell MC, Duncan GH, Hofbauer RK, Ha B, Chen JI, Carrier B. Pain perception: is there a role for primary somatosensory cortex?. *Proc Natl Acad Sci USA*. 1999;96:7705–7709.

221. Coghill RC, Sang CN, Maisog JM, Iadarola MJ. Pain intensity processing within the human brain: bilateral, distributed mechanism. *J Neurophysiol*. 1999;82:1934–1943.

222. Moulton EA, Keaser ML, Gullapalli RP, Greenspan JD. Regional intensive and temporal patterns of functional MRI activation distinguishing noxious and innocuous contact heat. *J Neurophysiol*. 2005;93:2183–2193.

223. Gustin SM, Wrigley PJ, Siddall PJ, Henderson LA. Brain anatomy changes associated with persistent neuropathic pain following spinal cord injury. *Cereb Cortex*. 2010;20:1409–1419.

224. Isokawa-Akesson M, Komisaruk BR. Difference in projections to the lateral and medial facial nucleus: anatomically separate pathways for rhythmical vibrissa movement in rats. *Exp Brain Res*. 1987;65:385–398.

225. Stanwell P, Siddall P, Keshava N, et al. Neuro magnetic resonance spectroscopy using wavelet decomposition and statistical testing identifies biochemical changes in people with spinal cord injury and pain. *Neuroimage*. 2010;53:544–552.

226. Paulson PE, Gorman AL, Yezierski RP, Casey KL, Morrow TJ. Differences in forebrain activation in two strains of rat at rest and after spinal cord injury. *Exp Neurol*. 2005;196:413–421.

227. Seminowicz DA, Jiang L, Ji Y, Xu S, Gullapalli RP, Masri R. Thalamocortical asynchrony in conditions of spinal cord injury pain in rats. *J Neurosci*. 2012;32:15843–15848.

228. Walton KD, Llinas RR. Central pain as a thalamocortical dysrhythmia: a thalamic efference disconnection?. In: Kruger L, Light AR, eds. *Translational Pain Research: From*

Mouse to Man. Boca Raton, FL: CRC Press; 2010. [Chapter 13. Available from: <http://www.ncbi.nlm.nih.gov/books/NBK57255/>.

229. Leznik E, Makarenko V, Llinas R. Electrotonically mediated oscillatory patterns in neuronal ensembles: an in vitro voltage-dependent dye-imaging study in the inferior olive. *J Neurosci.* 2002;22:2804–2815.

230. Llinas R, Urbano FJ, Leznik E, Ramirez RR, van Marle HJ. Rhythmic and dysrhythmic thalamocortical dynamics: GABA systems and the edge effect. *Trends Neurosci.* 2005;28:325–333.

231. Finnerup NB, Gottrup H, Jensen TS. Anticonvulsants in central pain. *Expert Opin Pharmacother.* 2002;3:1411–1420.

232. Namba S, Nakao Y, Matsumoto Y, Ohmoto T, Nishimoto A. Electrical stimulation of the posterior limb of the internal capsule for treatment of thalamic pain. *Appl Neurophysiol.* 1984;47:137–148.

233. Gybels J, Kupers R. Deep brain stimulation in the treatment of chronic pain in man: where and why?. *Neurophysiol Clin.* 1990;20:389–398.

234. Namba S, Nishimoto A. Stimulation of internal capsule, thalamic sensory nucleus (VPM) and cerebral cortex inhibited deafferentation hyperactivity provoked after gasserian ganglionectomy in cat. *Acta Neurochir Suppl (Wien).* 1988;42:243–247.

235. Tsubokawa T, Katayama Y, Yamamoto T, Hirayama T, Koyama S. Treatment of thalamic pain by chronic motor cortex stimulation. *Pacing Clin Electrophysiol.* 1991;14:131–134.

236. Brown JA, Pilitsis JG. Motor cortex stimulation for central and neuropathic facial pain: a prospective study of 10 patients and observations of enhanced sensory and motor function during stimulation. *Neurosurgery.* 2005;56:290–297. [discussion 290-7].

237. Ebel H, Rust D, Tronnier V, Boker D, Kunze S. Chronic precentral stimulation in trigeminal neuropathic pain. *Acta Neurochir (Wien).* 1996;138:1300–1306.

238. Sol JC, Casaux J, Roux FE, et al. Chronic motor cortex stimulation for phantom limb pain: correlations between pain relief and functional imaging studies. *Stereotact Funct Neurosurg.* 2001;77:172–176.

239. Boord P, Siddall PJ, Tran Y, Herbert D, Middleton J, Craig A. Electroencephalographic slowing and reduced reactivity in neuropathic pain following spinal cord injury. *Spinal Cord.* 2008;46:118–123.

240. Bezard E, Boraud T, Nguyen JP, Velasco F, Keravel Y, Gross C. Cortical stimulation and epileptic seizure: a study of the potential risk in primates. *Neurosurgery.* 1999;45:346–350.

241. Huang YZ, Edwards MJ, Rounis E, Bhatia KP, Rothwell JC. Theta burst stimulation of the human motor cortex. *Neuron.* 2005;45:201–206.

242. Fontaine D, Hamani C, Lozano A. Efficacy and safety of motor cortex stimulation for chronic neuropathic pain: critical review of the literature. *J Neurosurg.* 2009;110:251–256.

243. Lima MC, Fregni F. Motor cortex stimulation for chronic pain: systematic review and meta-analysis of the literature. *Neurology.* 2008;70:2329–2337.

244. Cruccu G. Treatment of painful neuropathy. *Curr Opin Neurol.* 2007;20:531–535.

245. Canavero S, Bonicalzi V. Central pain syndrome: elucidation of genesis and treatment. *Expert Rev Neurother.* 2007;7:1485–1497.

246. Peyron R, Faillenot I, Mertens P, Laurent B, Garcia-Larrea L. Motor cortex stimulation in neuropathic pain. Correlations between analgesic effect and hemodynamic changes in the brain. A PET study. *Neuroimage.* 2007;34:310–321.

247. Drouot X, Nguyen JP, Peschanski M, Lefaucheur JP. The antalgic efficacy of chronic motor cortex stimulation is related to sensory changes in the painful zone. *Brain.* 2002;125:1660–1664.

248. Lefaucheur JP, Drouot X, Menard-Lefaucheur I, Nguyen JP. Neuropathic pain controlled for more than a year by monthly sessions of repetitive transcranial magnetic stimulation of the motor cortex. *Neurophysiol Clin*. 2004;34:91–95.

249. Garcia-Larrea L, Peyron R. Motor cortex stimulation for neuropathic pain: from phenomenology to mechanisms. *Neuroimage*. 2007;37(suppl 1):S71–S79.

250. Garcia-Larrea L, Peyron R, Mertens P, et al. Positron emission tomography during motor cortex stimulation for pain control. *Stereotact Funct Neurosurg*. 1997;68:141–148.

251. Garcia-Larrea L, Peyron R, Mertens P, et al. Electrical stimulation of motor cortex for pain control: a combined PET-scan and electrophysiological study. *Pain*. 1999;83:259–273.

252. Schoenen J, Grant GS. Spinal cord: connections. In: Paxinos G, Mai JK, eds. *The Human Bervous System*. Amsterdam: Elsevier; 2004. p. 233–250.

253. Fonoff ET, Dale CS, Pagano RL, et al. Antinociception induced by epidural motor cortex stimulation in naive conscious rats is mediated by the opioid system. *Behav Brain Res*. 2009;196:63–70.

254. Viisanen H, Pertovaara A. Antinociception by motor cortex stimulation in the neuropathic rat: does the locus coeruleus play a role?. *Exp Brain Res*. 2010;201:283–296.

255. Tasker RR. Microelectrode findings in the thalamus in chronic pain and other conditions. *Stereotact Funct Neurosurg*. 2001;77:166–168.

256. Canavero S, Bonicalzi V. Cortical stimulation for central pain. *J Neurosurg*. 1995;83:1117.

257. Canavero S, Bonicalzi V, Castellano G, Perozzo P, Massa-Micon B. Painful supernumerary phantom arm following motor cortex stimulation for central poststroke pain. Case report. *J Neurosurg*. 1999;91:121–123.

258. Saitoh Y, Shibata M, Hirano S, Hirata M, Mashimo T, Yoshimine T. Motor cortex stimulation for central and peripheral deafferentation pain. Report of eight cases. *J Neurosurg*. 2000;92:150–155.

259. Canavero S, Bonicalzi V. Extradural cortical stimulation for movement disorders. *Acta Neurochir Suppl*. 2007;97:223–232.

260. Canavero S, Pagni CA, Castellano G, et al. The role of cortex in central pain syndromes: preliminary results of a long-term technetium-99 hexamethylpropyleneamineoxime single photon emission computed tomography study. *Neurosurgery*. 1993;32:185–189. [discussion 190-1].

261. Mitrofanis J, Mikuletic L. Organisation of the cortical projection to the zona incerta of the thalamus. *J Comp Neurol*. 1999;412:173–185.

262. Urbain N, Deschenês M. Motor cortex gates vibrissal responses in a thalamocortical projection pathway. *Neuron*. 2007;56:714–725.

263. Cha M, Ji Y, Masri R. Motor cortex stimulation activates the incertothalamic pathway in an animal model of spinal cord injury. *J Pain*. 2013 [in press].

7

Discussion

Carl Y. Saab

Brown University, Providence, RI, USA

SO WHAT'S NOVEL ABOUT THIS BOOK?

The concept of closely examining brain function with the aim of better understanding the underlying physiological mechanisms of pain is not new. However, the authors have strived to present up-to-date neurophysiological and imaging data, as well as state-of-the-art quantitative and computational methods to make sense of an increasingly complex set of information (for example functional connectivity between brain areas). In this sense, this book takes a *closer* look at brain mechanisms using relatively new techniques, as well as older tools used in novel ways.

More importantly, the empirical multidisciplinary evidence presented here leverages basic science and clinical data with practical solutions (such as potential diagnostic, therapeutic and device technology) in a field where major translational breakthroughs have been largely unimpressive for the past few decades. Namely, the increasing spatial resolution of imaging is allowing researchers to pin-point regions of interest in the brain, with intricate anatomical precision, that are showing abnormal functional and anatomical abnormalities in pain patients. In parallel, neurophysiological techniques, ranging from single units, to simultaneous recordings of hundreds of units with multichannel electrode arrays, to local field potentials, to EEG, to MEG, are making it possible to ask what exactly is going on in these regions of interest at the cellular and circuitry levels? Laboratory animal models are further allowing us to interrogate and to directly manipulate brain circuitry in ways that are not yet feasible or ethically permissible in human subjects. These cross-disciplinary efforts are finally informing theoretical researchers in formulating and fine-tuning experimentally falsifiable claims.

IN DEFENSE OF STUDYING THE BRAIN

Going back to the idea of why focus on the brain, instead of for e.g. the spinal cord or peripheral nerves, though the rationale in favor of our approach has been defended in Introduction based on scientific and philosophical grounds, I would add that 1) particular cases of chronic pain secondary to thalamic syndrome or migraine represent straightforward and strong arguments for referring the condition in question to a disorder in brain function, such that exploring spinal cord and peripheral circuitries would resemble embarking on an expedition to the West Pole, 2) it is very reasonable to study the cognitive and emotive correlates of pain by studying brain function 3) unequivocal evidence suggests that distinct brain mechanisms have the power to directly modulate pain experiences, such as mirror therapy for phantom limb pain (discussed below in more detail) and visual of the modulation perception of experimental and moderately noxious stimuli. For example, individuals asked to look at their hand while it is being subjected to an infrared laser stimulus report less intense pain compared to when they are looking away at another object, suggesting that active recruitment of visual brain circuits can reduce the experience of acute pain.[1]

A corollary, albeit important, claim in the book is that research into the mechanisms of chronic pain in the brain is essentially a neuroscientific inquiry. This is especially true, as far as the techniques used to answer questions relevant to brain function are empirically measurable using *neuro*imaging or *neuro*physiological tools. In this sense, we leave the conceptual entanglement regarding "language games" (for example epistemology and ontology of pain) to the domain of *neuro*-philosophy (a burgeoning field not necessarily orthogonal in interests to mainstream neuroscience) or spirituality (for example yoga and hypnotism).

TO IMAGE A WHOLE BRAIN, NOT JUST ITS PARTS

A common trap in which most pain researchers fall into is the reduction of experimentally-evoked pain to a point in time typically in the order of few milliseconds preceding and following an applied noxious stimulus. Furthermore, many pain researchers would prefer to confine pain-related signals to a restricted anatomical locus in the brain. However, human experiences signaling physical harm engage a system of memories and believes, while calling into play a set of action plans to mitigate the threat. This complicated, yet cohesive and comprehensive response transcends the one second timeframe arbitrarily imposed by many studies investigating pain-evoked brain activity. Human beings have evolved beyond the reflexive pattern of movements towards an intelligent behavior accompanied with enough emotional and cognitive maturity to guide us through safety, and, most importantly, to allow us to interpret and communicate danger signals and evasion tactics to our offspring and community.

Therefore, painful episodes trigger *intelligent* responses sometimes lasting minutes, hours, or even a lifetime, depending on severity. Such an intelligent design of the pain system is based on the brain's machinery and is restricted by the physical and biological laws governing brain function. However, when considering that the "processing speed" of neurons is in the order of 100 Hz, which is about 7 orders of magnitude slower than the time it takes vacuum tubes and transistors to perform logical operations in household "smart" devices ($\sim10^9$ s), one wonders how does the brain compensate for such a disadvantage? In contrast to the digital and serial computational models of computers, a human brain with all its allegedly 10^{14} synaptic connections functions like an analogue parallel processor able to perform $10^2 \times 10^{14}$ operations *simultaneously*, at least hypothetically. Considering the complexity of the human experience of, and response to, pain, it is very likely that the pain-related brain activity is widespread spatially and temporally. It is rather peculiar that the imaging community studying pain has just recently shifted towards what it considered as a *novel* paradigm for analyzing fMRI voxels using multivariate statistics.

Simply put, multivariate pattern analysis (MVPA) uses a classification algorithm to decode information in spatially distributed multi-voxels simultaneously.[2,3] According to MVPA, a classifier is trained to predict the nth state of mind (for e.g. pain *versus* no-pain) from known n^{th-1} preceding states using linear support vector machine (SVM) learning. Though this approach has been described as a breakthrough in fMRI pain and cognition-related studies, it is hardly a new concept. Here's what Paul and Patricia Churchland had to say in their preface to the second edition of von Neumann's book "The Computer and the Brain"[4]:

> The alternative computational strategy on which von Neumann speculated now appears to be an instance of the simultaneous multiplication of each of many thousands or millions of simultaneous axonal spiking frequencies (which constitute a very large *input vector*) by the coefficients of an even larger matrix (namely, the configuration of the many millions of synaptic junctions that connect one neuronal population to the next) to produce an *output vector*. It is the acquired global configuration of those many millions, nay trillions, of synaptic connections that embodies whatever knowledge and skills the brain may have acquired.

It is quite revealing that these statements made in the year 2000 (commenting on a book written in 1958) explicitly use the words "vector" and "matrix" which are currently being hailed as innovative in the pain imaging literature.

The Sensory Field Lags Behind the Motor Field

In the history of neuroscience, studies related to the motor system have superceded those of the sensory system. A basic proof-of-principle experiment for the nerve conduction hypothesis is dramatically illustrated in the early works of Luigi Galvani who showed in the late eighteenth century that electrical stimulation of the sciatic nerve resulted in muscular contraction of a dead frog's hind limb. This observation made Galvani the first to appreciate the relationship between electricity and animation and provided the basis for electrical energy underlying movement. This discovery laid down to rest the Cartesian theory of "animal spirits" running down wires to initiate movement proposed more than a century earlier.

Since then, the most influential neuroscientists of our time, including Sherrington and Eccles, have tackled core physiological concepts predominantly relevant to the motor nervous system, such as reflexes. It appears as though the tradition of favoring the motor system has endured, perhaps at the expense of the sensory system. Here we are, more than two centuries after the dead frog experiment and fast forward to the world of brain-machine-interfaces for restoring movement in paralyzed limbs, still entrapped in language games regarding sensory experiences, unable to come to grips with a phenomenon that is not amenable to quantitative measurements (sensation cannot be shown with the same ease as movements), completely ignorant of the neural basis for the genealogy of sensory experiences, and frustrated by our incapacity to effectively treat and manage chronic pain and other sensory disorders.

Let's briefly entertain extreme cases of motor and sensory deficits (for example paralysis and anesthesia) and in-between cases of less extreme motor and sensory disorders (for example tremors and dysesthesias). It is obvious that patients with motor disturbances have more and better choices than their counterparts with sensory disturbances. Even patients in a vegetative state can now make use of novel technologies that allow for their control of a robotic arm at will.[5] It is also pretty impressive that the neocortical circuitry for some motor areas have been exquisitely mapped so that simple grasp movements of the arm can be modeled mathematically, based on the activity of less than 100 neurons, to predict the position and velocity of the hand and arm with almost 95% accuracy.[6] The same cannot be said with regards to our understanding of the neocortical substrates of sensory experiences. Parkinsonian patients have multiple choices including pharmacotherapy (levodopa, a revolutionary therapy in neurology) and highly effective deep brain stimulation. Again, the same does not hold true for pain patients or those with severe dysesthesia. One is inclined to ask whether any of these strategies used to better understand and treat disorders of the motor system are valid, useful and adaptable for the sensory system?

No Rigid Sensory/Motor Dichotomy in Pain Research

The strict dichotomy between motor and sensory systems in pain research should be dropped. At least two counterexamples come to mind in support of a more liberal approach to studying the pain system. First is the body of evidence showing major nociceptive input to the cerebellum in humans and animal subjects, as well as the capacity of the cerebellum to modulate nociceptive reflexes, at least under experimental conditions. Indeed, Patrick Wall eloquently argued:

> There are elaborate and extensive areas of our brain concerned with motor planning as distinct from motor movement itself. It is precisely these areas that are most active when the brain is imaged in subjects who are in pain but who are quite stationary with no movement. [...] I am proposing a quite new hypothesis here, one should explore widely to see if there are facts which support the possibility that sensory analysis is carried on in terms of motor action which would be appropriate to the input. [...] The marked activation of the cerebellum is a great surprise because classical opinion assigned no sensory role to the cerebellum. However, more recent work has clearly shown that the cerebellum plays a role in the analysis of sensory input in the course of establishing responses (p. 3).[7]

We now know that the cerebellum, traditionally considered a "motor" brain region, is consistently reported to be activated in pain imaging studies; however, no valid explanation is usually offered to justify its role in the sensory/emotive experience of pain, if any.

The cerebellum is an integrator of motor and sensory processes. Maps of cerebellar activity that encode tactile vibratory stimulation as well as movement of the fingers largely overlap,[8] and further support the fractured somatotopic organization of the cerebellar cortex. Parallel experiments also show increased cerebellar activity during nociceptive and aversive events, such as noxious heat and passive viewing of unpleasant images in humans,[9–11] as well as intradermal hindpaw injection of capsaicin in rats (Saab, 2000). Activity of cerebellar Purkinje cells is modulated by noxious somatic and visceral stimuli.[12] Interestingly, electrical stimulation of the cerebellar cortical vermis enhances, whereas stimulation of the fastigial cerebellar nucleus attenuates, nociceptive visceromotor reflexes in the rat.[13] Cerebellar cortical stimulation also increases the firing of visceroceptive lumbosacral neurons to colorectal distension, with a variable modulatory effect on the responses of these cells to somatic stimuli.[14] Another laboratory has followed-up on these experiments in recent days, showing that electrical stimulation using electrodes inserted 1 mm below the surface of the intermediate hemisphere of the anterior cerebellar cortex reduces nociceptive responses of spinal cord dorsal horn neurons.[15] However, with respect to the exceptionally high voltage used in these experiments (>10 V), it is difficult to ascertain whether stimulation involved cerebellar cortical and/or nuclear structures, even reaching non-cerebellar structures. Therefore, it is conceivable that the cerebellum may modulate adaptive motor control of nociceptive reflexes, as well as perhaps emotive and cognitive responses to pain, as has been speculated.[11]

The second counterexample is the emerging evidence for the analgesic effect of electrical stimulation in the motor cortex (see Chapter 6 in this book by Keller and Masri).

With regards to voluntary movement, how will/thought leads to action remains enigmatic. However, researchers are inching closer to identifying the neural substrate in the neocortex of relatively simple movements at the molecular, cellular, circuitry, ensembles and maps levels, extending all the way to emergent properties. The brain (mainly neocortex) is faced with solving the problem of motor plan and execution. Several areas are known to be linked to the motor cortex, however, as discussed previously, grasp motion of the hand can be decoded with 95% accuracy based on multiple unit activity of less than 100 neurons in the motor cortex,[6] suggesting that these other brain areas contribute for full accuracy and precision (not withstanding possible redundancy in the system). Though maps of the motor homunculus turned out to be more plastic than originally depicted by Wilder Penfield, it remains that targeted stimulation of specific areas can evoke motor responses (at least muscle twitches) in corresponding body parts, whereas sensory maps seem more elusive based on a similar strategy. Moreover, the task of decoding neuronal ensembles that control hand grasp is made easier by the fact that the motor output can be finely captured and measured in time and space, whereas the same cannot be said regarding sensory experiences. Finally, the entire motor system down-stream from the neocortex can be by-passed all together in the case of paralysis, so that brain-machine-interface devices can directly transform neuronal output from the motor cortex to a motor command in a machine. Evidently, the same is not applicable in the case of sensory deficits and non-sensical in the case of chronic pain.

The Old, the New and the Re-Furbished Neuromodulation Techniques

Regardless of the polemic relationship between brain mechanisms and sensory experiences (causality *versus* correlation), the fact remains that modulation of brain activity by pharmaceutical, cognitive, genetic or technological means can have a significant impact on brain function and, consequently, cognition in general. Therefore, one can safely entertain the idea that neuromodulation constitutes a valid rationale for therapeutic interventions in the case of cognitive and/or sensory disorders, including pain. The targets and modes of action of drug-based therapies in the CNS for pain management has been well-discussed elsewhere,[7,16] therefore, in this section, only technological approaches targeting the brain will be discussed, including electrical, optogenetic and ultrasonic neuromodulation techniques.

Up until approximately half a decade ago, the tools available to neuroscientists for interrogating the functional circuitry of the nervous system consisted almost exclusively of electrical, magnetic, and photonic-based methods. Traditionally, electrical stimulation of nervous tissue reigned supreme over all other techniques of neuromodulation. The major concerns on everybody's mind looking to stimulate or silence neurons in the brain include safety and specificity. Issues related to safety take on different levels of severity ranging from none in the case of *in vitro* preparations, to moderate in laboratory settings using non-human primates or rodents, to considerable (but not insurmountable) worries in a clinical environment. Other concerns, on the other hand, revolve around achieving optimal spatial and temporal resolutions, while leveraging specificity. Researchers often rank neuromodulation techniques based on these constraints weighed against the degrees of freedom allowed by the experimental design in question.

Readers interested in a comprehensive and up-to-date discussion of neuromodulation are referred to *Neuromodulation*, an authoritative two-volume textbook written by leading experts in the field. In that book, neuromodulation is defined as "technology impacting on the neuronal interface. It is the process of inhibition, stimulation, modification, regulation or therapeutic alteration of activity, electrically or chemically, in the central, peripheral or autonomic nervous system. It is the science of how electrical, chemical, and mechanical interventions can modulate the nervous system function" (p. 3).[17] With regards to the use of electrical neuromodulation for pain, the book recounts a story that "a freed slave of Emperor Tiberius was suffering from painful gout. He accidentally stepped on an electric torpedo fish and suffered a sudden severe shock. Afterward, he had much less gout pain. The Emperor's physician, Scribonius, write that thereafter he recommended the torpedo fish treatment for chronically persistent pain".[18]

Neuromodulation by Electricity

Deep brain stimulation (DBS) is considered primarily a neurosurgical intervention intended to manage severe intractable pain. Although the safety and efficacy of DBS were established firmly for movement disorders, DBS for pain remains "off-label" and its mechanisms remain largely unknown. In general, the primary disadvantage of using electrodes is the requirement for surgical procedures, with the potential to trigger inflammation, cell death and gliosis cascades.[19] The main targets of DBS for pain include thalamic and brain stem structures. Current indications include pain secondary to stroke, amputation (phantom pain), failed back surgeries and cancer, thus mainly of neuropathic origin. Interestingly, the frequencies used during DBS for pain range typically from 50–70 Hz (see discussion below regarding low- versus high-frequency stimulation).

Today, conventional wisdom equates "electrical stimulation" with "neuronal excitation," but it is becoming increasingly clear that different electrical stimulation parameters may result in gain or loss of function in a neuronal population exposed to a *stimulating* probe. For example, though the mechanisms of DBS remain speculative,[20] studies related to DBS for motor disorders suggest that high-frequency stimulation (HFS, >100 Hz) can mimic the functional effects of ablation,[21] also referred to as "jamming" of neuronal circuitry.[20] In animal models, two studies have recently tested the effects of deep brain stimulation (DBS) on sensitization of single-units in the brain, as well as on pain behavior.[22,23] Aiming to reverse neuronal sensitization in the sensory ventral posterolateral (VPL) nucleus of the thalamus, HFS (100–150 Hz) within the VPL was shown to effectively decrease neuronal hyperexcitability and thermal hyperalgesia in an animal model of peripheral pain, whereas stimulation at a low-frequency (LFS, 20–40 Hz) had no effect on neuronal firing.[22] Interestingly, LFS (50 Hz) in the VPL is known to produce little or no analgesia in rats.[24] In another animal model of central pain, LFS (50 Hz) within the motor cortex reduced mechanical allodynia and thermal hyperalgesia.[23] These effects were shown to be mimicked by DBS in the zona incerta of the subthalamus and blocked by reversible inactivation of this region (see Chapter 6 in this book by Keller and Masri). This suggests that the potential analgesic effects of motor cortex stimulation may be due to disinhibition of the zona incerta, thus, causing analgesia by restoring inhibition in the thalamus.

In parallel to the effects of DBS detailed above at the single-cell level, there is a possibility that DBS may modulate network function at the level of the local field potential (LFP), mainly oscillations at the low-frequency end of the EEG spectrum (<30 Hz). Indeed, analgesic efficacy of DBS in the VPL/VPM is positively correlated with LFP amplitude,[25,26] whereas chronic pain patients manifest enhanced LFP power spectra in the low frequency range (8–15 Hz) of PVG/PAG and VPL/VPM. Intraoperative recordings of cortical LFPs have been used in humans subjected to cutaneous application of a moderately noxious laser stimulus. Though invasive, this technique was shown to be useful for analyzing the directional and temporal dynamics within- and between-cortical structures in awake subjects combined with Granger causality method,[27,28] suggesting that S1 cortex may be the primary drive for activity in other parts of the pain matrix (also see Chapter 3 in this book by Markman et al.).

By comparison to intracranial recording, there is preference for the use of non-invasive techniques as biomarkers for pain, such as EEG[29] and MEG techniques that could be used for the analysis of oscillatory components of LFPs. When resting EEG is compared between healthy subjects and patients with neurogenic pain, a significantly higher spectral power is detected in patients over the frequency range 2–25 Hz with a leftward shift of the dominant median peak.[30] Therapeutic lesion in the thalamus (central lateral nucleus) of these patients significantly reduces pain within 12 months after surgery and decreases the average EEG power in the theta band approaching normal values. This suggests that both EEG and pain are determined by tightly coupled brain mechanisms, presumably mediated by thalamocortical loops. In another similar study, enhanced EEG power spectra was reported in the high theta (6–9 Hz) and low beta frequency ranges (12–16 Hz) and localized to pain-associated cortical areas including the insula, cingulate cortex, PFC, and S1.[31] Using MEG, a leftward 2–3 Hz shift from the normal range of 8–10 Hz was reported in the median dominant spectral power of patients with complex regional pain syndrome.[32] In general, MEG has long been postulated to reveal abnormal theta range spectral power in patients with different cognitive disorders, such as schizophrenia and obsessive-compulsive disorders[32,33] (also see Chapter 4 in this book by Llinas and Walton).

Accordingly, it is envisioned that neuromodulation of brain activity can be optimized when guided by empirical evidence from a variety of imaging and/or electrophysiological techniques. Neuromodulation for the direct inhibition of neuronal activity in hyperactive brain regions is proposed as an alternative to traditional approaches involving stimulation of descending analgesic systems or the ascending spinal cord dorsal column system, which are thought to produce analgesic effects indirectly. Importantly, effects of the various neuromodulation techniques on glial cells need to be studied in more detail. For example, astrocytic calcium signaling in the hippocampus has been demonstrated to be critical for cholinergic-induced synaptic plasticity and long-term potentiation,[34] thus, are likely to be important in neuronal plasticity related to long-term nociception.

Other forms of electrical stimulation not requiring invasive surgical procedures for access to the stimulation site include electroconvulsive shock *therapy* (with questionable therapeutic benefit), and the more tolerated transcranial direct current stimulation (tDCS) and transcranial magnetic stimulation (TMS). As opposed to the "whole sale" and very diffuse effects of electroconvulsive shock, the spatial resolution within the brain parenchyma for tDCS and TMS through intact rodent or primate skull can reach one or few centimeters, which is till considerably larger compared to microelectrode stimulation in the order of hundred of micrometers or a few millimeters range, depending on stimulation parameters and microelectrode properties. Both tDCS and TMS have been successfully shown to stimulate intact cortical and subcortical tissue,[35,36,37,38,39] whereas TMS has been recently approved by the FDA for the treatment of depressive mood disorders (Horvath, Mathews et al.). Though all methods based on electrical stimulation (or magnetic fields generating inductive electrical charges) offer exquisite temporal resolutions, they remain non-specific with regards to the types of neuronal and glial cells stimulated and their cellular processes (i.e. axons and dendrites).

Neuromodulation by Sound

Transcranial pulsed ultrasound (TPU) is a novel technique that generates acoustic pressure waves through the intact skull, thus functionally activating a non-specific group of cells within the brain with an estimated lateral spatial resolution in the order of a couple millimeters.[40,41] Motor cortical activation using TPU evokes motor behavior in mice, whereas activation in the hippocampus triggers synchronous oscillations.[41] Though the exact mechanisms of action of TPU are incompletely understood, it is speculated that the mechanical waves generated by ultrasound waves can excite cells by adiabatical propagation through neuronal membranes. For example, ultrasound waves propagation in lipid membranes produce depolarizing potentials between 1–50 mV with insignificant heat generation.[42] Similarly, ultrasound waves may depolarize neuronal membranes above firing threshold by activating voltage-gated ion channels. However, waves are also capable of tissue ablation by causing cavitational damage, typically at pressures >40 MPa. Indeed, magnetic resonance-guided focused ultrasound (MRgFUS) has been successfully used to perform non-invasive thalamotomies with millimeter accuracy for the treatment of intractable chronic pain.[43] It is important to note that at peak rarefactional pressures <1 MPa, ultrasound has been reported to be effective in stimulating brain tissue in mice with no damage at cellular, histological, ultrastructural and behavioral levels.[41,44] Implementation of hyperlenses and acoustic metamaterials for focusing ultrasound waves might enable enhancement of subdiffraction-limited spatial resolutions in the near future.[40]

Neuromodulation by Light: Key to Solving Population Coding

While the vast majority of studies investigating neuronal brain function of pain patients and animal models are based on single unit activity, there is emerging evidence that LFPs carry significant information content, including the processing of nociceptive information. Historically, when the broad tuning of individual neurons cannot account for the discriminative ability of the system in question, the concept of population coding comes to mind. As James McIlwain succinctly put it, "a 'signature' of a system that employs a distributed code is that its neurons taken one at a time are broadly tuned along a dimension that the system nonetheless appears to resolve with a high degree of precision".[45] Take for example wide dynamic range neurons that respond to non-noxious peripheral touch, as well as to pinch and thermal stimuli with an almost ubiquitous increased rate of firing, yet our sensory experiences of each of these modalities is quite distinct. A major problem, though, has been that probing neuronal circuitry using electricity or less-traditional ultrasound techniques lack the cellular specificity for highly selective targeting of neurons in the brain, until recently.

With regards to rhythmic oscillation, one of the strongest cases for the importance of a specific cell type in rhythmic oscillation is the role of fast-spiking (FS) interneurons in gamma oscillations. Networks of FS neurons connected by gap junctions provide synchronous inhibitory post-synaptic potentials (IPSP) to local excitatory neurons. Indeed, pyramidal excitatory neurons are thought to be entrained to the rhythmic inhibitory activity.[46,47] Using optogenetic tools, it was recently possible to test this hypothesis by selectively activating FS interneurons in barrel cortex at varied frequencies, thereby amplifying gamma oscillations, whereas pyramidal neuron activation amplified only lower frequency oscillations in a cell-type-specific double dissociation paradigm.[48] The authors of that study further concluded that distinct network activity states can be induced in vivo by selective targeting of specific cell population.

How does optogenetic manipulation work? You basically need a light source to shine on a population of neurons expressing a light-sensitive membrane channel. Stimulation selectivity is conferred by the exclusive expression of these membrane channels within a sub-population of neurons, usually using genetic approaches. In practical terms, various cascades of genes were first tested as multicomponent approaches for optical control, such as rhodopsin and arrestin genes from Drosophila photoreceptors were combined to light-sensitive neurons. Later, single-component approaches such as microbial opsin methods were introduced for light-induced inward cation currents, causing depolarization of neuronal membranes and positively modulating action potential firing (Fenno, Yizhar et al.). To date, there are several optogenetic tools optimized for neuronal excitation (using channelrhodopsin-1, ChR1 or ChR2, blue-light-activated nonspecific cation channels), neuronal inhibition (using halorhodopsin NpHR derived from *Natronomonas pharaonis*), biochemical control (using GPCRs converted into light-sensitive regulators of intracellular signaling pathways or OptoXRs), developmental and layer-specific targeting, as well as circuit targeting (for further details refer to (Fenno, Yizhar et al.). The animal models amenable to optogenetic manipulation are diverse, including *Caenorhabditis elegans*, fly, zebrafish, mouse, rat, and non-human primate.

The use of transgenic or knock-in animals offers the added benefit of tighter control of transgene expression, bypassing other viral modes of transfection of genes coding for light-sensitive channels. However, these strategies are not perfect and are still undergoing constant improvements, for example on-going efforts to address the inherent limitation of the ChR2 system whose temporal precision is compromised by a relatively extended deactivation time constant (10–12 ms) upon cessation of light. Nevertheless, optogenetic tools can achieve specific neuronal excitation or inhibition *in vitro* and in freely moving animals, allowing for the control of neuronal activity at an exceedingly high temporal scale. Implementation of optogenetic manipulation in non-human primates and in humans, however, has been more challenging.

Neuromodulation by Visual Cues: The Vietnam-Cambodia Mirror Therapy Project

Ditch the pill and the high-cost techniques, bring a mirror and let us explore a virtually zero-cost, groundbreaking therapy for a mysterious form of chronic pain classified as phantom pain. That's the journey that a team of researchers embarked on, by launching a training project introduced first in Vietnam in 2011 (as a collaboration between Beth Darnall, PhD, of Oregon, Health and Science University and Moira Judith Mann, co-founder of the End the Pain Project), and soon thereafter expanded to neighboring Cambodia this year. Joining forces with Do Than Huy, MSC, MA, Chief of Anesthesiology, Can Tho University, and Tuan Ahn Nguyen, MMed, of University Medical Center in Ho Chi Minh City, Darnall and Mann received a grant from the International Association for the Study of Pain under the Initiative for Improving Pain Education in Developing Countries.[49] The project's aim was primarily to fund training in mirror therapy to local physicians, trauma workers, physical therapists, prosthetists, and allied health professionals. Vietnam is a country of limited resources with exceedingly high prevalence of amputation secondary to landmines and motorbike accidents.

In Cambodia, for example, the first part of the workshop consisted of involving volunteer amputees with phantom pain and guiding them through a mirror therapy session. In the second part, physiotherapists and prosthetists self-administered the therapy, experiencing sensations caused by concentrating on mirror images of their limbs in simple motion exercises.

The study suggests that mirror therapy procedures can be taught to amputees, whom up to 80% experience phantom pain, in less than an hour by a trained professional. Thus, it is astounding that badly needed self-treatment that is simple, completely safe, non-invasive and non-addictive can be contemplated conveniently in a home setting using a relatively inexpensive and accessible device: mirror! At the end of the study, 106 workshop participants received certificates of completion with satisfaction ratings reaching 96%. Statistical t-test further confirmed significantly greater likelihood to use mirror therapy with future patients.

SELF-CRITIQUE OF A PAIN NEUROSCIENTIST

As a neuroscientist by training, I'm inclined to compare between the state of the art in the field of brain research, including the brilliant work being done to understand and treat epilepsy, movement disorders and Alzheimer's *versus* the pain field. Some might inevitably disagree with the following statement, but the facts show that the pain arena is lagging tremendously behind its counterparts in CNS disorders. One has to ask: Are we taking an irrational approach, asking the wrong questions (searching for "pain centers," using the wrong tools, facing crippling regulatory constraints, or bugged down by social stigma from the lobotomy era? I hope at least modestly that this book has succeeded in identifying areas of strengths in pain research, pitfalls and promising visions for future neuroscientists, not just those in the microbiology and electrophysiology trenches, but also computational "geeks" standing at the interface between man-machine to inspire the next-generation. In the end, only a genuine open source collaborative effort will yield reliable diagnostic biomarkers and safe therapy for pain. Such breakthroughs may potentially have spill over effects to cognitive and psychiatric disorders that have been thus far intractable or only tractable by traditional pharmacotherapy.

References

1. Longo MR, Gian Domenico Iannetti Thinking pain and the body: neural correlates of visually induced Analgesia. *J Neurosci.* 2012
2. Brodersen KH, Wiech K, et al. Decoding the perception of pain from fMRI using multivariate pattern analysis. *Neuroimage.* 2012;63(3):1162–1170.
3. Schulz E, Tiemann L, et al. Gamma oscillations are involved in the sensorimotor transformation of pain.. *J Neurophysiol.* 2012;108(4):1025–1031.
4. Neumann Jv. *The Computer and the Brain.* New Haven: Yale University Press; 1958.
5. Hochberg LR, Serruya MD, et al. Neuronal ensemble control of prosthetic devices by a human with tetraplegia. *Nature.* 2006;442(7099):164–171.

6. Bansal AK, Truccolo W, et al. Decoding 3D reach and grasp from hybrid signals in motor and premotor cortices: spikes, multiunit activity, and local field potentials. *J Neurophysiol*. 2012;107(5):1337–1355.

7. Wall PD. *Textbook of Pain*. New York: Churchill Livingstone; 1999.

8. Wiestler T, McGonigle DJ, et al. Integration of sensory and motor representations of single fingers in the human cerebellum. *J Neurophysiol*. 2011;105(6):3042–3053.

9. Moulton EA, Elman I, et al. Aversion-related circuitry in the cerebellum: responses to noxious heat and unpleasant images. *J Neurosci*. 2011;31(10):3795–3804.

10. Moulton EA, Pendse G, et al. BOLD responses in somatosensory cortices better reflect heat sensation than pain. *J Neurosci*. 2012;32(17):6024–6031.

11. Moulton EA, Schmahmann JD, et al. The cerebellum and pain: passive integrator or active participator?. *Brain Res Rev*. 2010;65(1):14–27.

12. Saab CY, Willis WD. The cerebellum: organization, functions and its role in nociception. *Brain Res Brain Res Rev*. 2003;42(1):85–95.

13. Saab CY, Willis WD. Cerebellar stimulation modulates the intensity of a visceral nociceptive reflex in the rat. *Exp Brain Res*. 2002;146(1):117–121.

14. Saab CY, Willis WD. Nociceptive visceral stimulation modulates the activity of cerebellar Purkinje cells. *Exp Brain Res*. 2001;140(1):122–126.

15. Hagains CE, Senapati AK, et al. Inhibition of spinal cord dorsal horn neuronal activity by electrical stimulation of the cerebellar cortex. *J Neurophysiol*. 2011

16. Dworkin RH, Turk DC, et al. Evidence-based clinical trial design for chronic pain pharmacotherapy: a blueprint for ACTION. *Pain*. 2011;152(3 Suppl):S107–S115.

17. Krames ES, Peckham PH, et al. *Neuromodulation*. New York: Elsevier; 2009.

18. Stillings D. *The First use of Electricity for Pain Treatment*. Minnesota: Medtronic Inc; 1971.

19. Grill WM, Norman SE, et al. Implanted neural interfaces: biochallenges and engineered solutions. *Annu Rev Biomed Eng*. 2009;11:1–24.

20. Benabid AL, Benazzous A, et al. Mechanisms of deep brain stimulation. *Mov Disord*. 2002;17(Suppl 3):S73–S74.

21. Hammond C, Ammari R, et al. Latest view on the mechanism of action of deep brain stimulation. *Mov Disord*. 2008;23(15):2111–2121.

22. Iwata M, Leblanc BW, et al. High-frequency stimulation in the ventral posterolateral thalamus reverses electrophysiologic changes and hyperalgesia in a rat model of peripheral neuropathic pain. *Pain*. 2011;52(11):2505–2513.

23. Lucas JM, Ji Y, et al. Motor cortex stimulation reduces hyperalgesia in an animal model of central pain. *Pain*. 2011;152(6):1398–1407.

24. Mayer DJ, Liebeskind JC. Pain reduction by focal electrical stimulation of the brain: an anatomical and behavioral analysis. *Brain Res*. 1974;68(1):73–93.

25. Nandi D, Aziz T, et al. Thalamic field potentials in chronic central pain treated by periventricular gray stimulation—a series of eight cases. *Pain*. 2003;101(1-2):97–107.

26. Nandi D, Liu X, et al. Thalamic field potentials during deep brain stimulation of periventricular gray in chronic pain. *Pain*. 2002;97(1-2):47–51.

27. Liu CC, Franaszczuk P, et al. Studies of properties of 'Pain Networks' as predictors of targets of stimulation for treatment of pain. *Front Integr Neurosci*. 2011;5:80.

28. Liu CC, Ohara S, et al. Attention to painful cutaneous laser stimuli evokes directed functional connectivity between activity recorded directly from human pain-related cortical structures. *Pain*. 2011;152(3):664–675.

29. Prichep LS, John ER, et al. Evaluation of the pain matrix using EEG source localization: a feasibility study. *Pain Med*. 2011;12(8):1241–1248.

30. Sarnthein J, Stern J, et al. Increased EEG power and slowed dominant frequency in patients with neurogenic pain. *Brain*. 2006;129(Pt 1):55–64.

31. Stern J, Jeanmonod D, et al. Persistent EEG overactivation in the cortical pain matrix of neurogenic pain patients. *NeuroImage*. 2006;31(2):721–731.

32. Walton KD, Dubois M, et al. Abnormal thalamocortical activity in patients with Complex Regional Pain Syndrome (CRPS) type I. *Pain*. 2010;150(1):41–51.
33. Schulman JJ, Cancro R, et al. Imaging of thalamocortical dysrhythmia in neuropsychiatry. *Front Hum Neurosci*. 2011;5:69.
34. Navarrete M, Perea G, et al. Astrocytes mediate in vivo cholinergic-induced synaptic plasticity. *PLoS Biol*. 2012;10(2):e1001259.
35. Boggio PS, Nunes A, et al. Repeated sessions of noninvasive brain DC stimulation is associated with motor function improvement in stroke patients. *Restor Neurol Neurosci*. 2007;25(2):123–129.
36. Fregni F, Pascual-Leone A. Technology insight: noninvasive brain stimulation in neurology-perspectives on the therapeutic potential of rTMS and tDCS. *Nat Clin Pract Neurol*. 2007;3(7):383–393.
37. Haghighi SS. Transcranial stimulation parameters to elicit motor evoked potentials.. *Electromyogr Clin Neurophysiol*. 2006;46(7-8):409–412.
38. Wagner T, Valero-Cabre A, et al. Noninvasive human brain stimulation. *Annu Rev Biomed Eng*. 2007;9:527–565.
39. Zhang YP, Shields LB, et al. Use of magnetic stimulation to elicit motor evoked potentials, somatosensory evoked potentials, and H-reflexes in non-sedated rodents. *J Neurosci Methods*. 2007;165(1):9–17.
40. Tufail Y, Yoshihiro A, et al. Ultrasonic neuromodulation by brain stimulation with transcranial ultrasound. *Nat Protoc*. 2011;6(9):1453–1470.
41. Tyler WJ, Tufail Y, et al. Remote excitation of neuronal circuits using low-intensity, low-frequency ultrasound. *PLoS One*. 2008;3(10):e3511.
42. Griesbauer J, Wixforth A, et al. Wave propagation in lipid monolayers. *Biophys J*. 2009;97(10):2710–2716.
43. Martin E, Jeanmonod D, et al. High-intensity focused ultrasound for noninvasive functional neurosurgery. *Ann Neurol*. 2009;66(6):858–861.
44. Tufail Y, Matyushov A, et al. Transcranial pulsed ultrasound stimulates intact brain circuits. *Neuron*. 2010;66(5):681–694.
45. McIlwain JT. Population coding: a historical sketch. *Prog Brain Res*. 2001;130:3–7.
46. Whittington MA, Traub RD, et al. Recurrent excitatory postsynaptic potentials induced by synchronized fast cortical oscillations. *Proc Natl Acad Sci U S A*. 1997;94(22):12198–12203.
47. Whittington MA, Traub RD, et al. Synchronized oscillations in interneuron networks driven by metabotropic glutamate receptor activation. *Nature*. 1995;373(6515):612–615.
48. Cardin JA, Carlen M, et al. Driving fast-spiking cells induces gamma rhythm and controls sensory responses. *Nature*. 2009;459(7247):663–667.
49. IASP *IASP Insight*. 2012;1(1):2.

Index

Note: Page numbers followed by *"f"* and *"t"* refer to figures and tables, respectively.

I

IASP. *See* International Association for the Study of Pain (IASP)

IBS. *See* Irritable bowel syndrome (IBS)

Inhibitory post-synaptic potentials (IPSP), 48, 137

Insular cortex, 75–76

International Association for the Study of Pain (IASP), 2–3, 138

Interspike intervals (ISIs), 48

Intrathecal opioids, 81–82

IPSP. *See* Inhibitory post-synaptic potentials (IPSP)

Irritable bowel syndrome (IBS), 25–26

ISIs. *See* Interspike intervals (ISIs)

L

Laser evoked potentials (LEPs), 43

LEP. *See* Laser evoked potentials (LEPs)

Leprosy, 4–5

Location, of pain, 11

Low threshold spike (LTS), 46, 48

LTS. *See* Low threshold spike (LTS)

M

Magnetic resonance-guided focused ultrasound (MRgFUS), 136

Magnetoencephalography (MEG)
power spectra and localization, 64–65
power spectra and sources of theta activity, 62–63
techniques, 42

Maladaptive plasticity, 95–96, 100, 103–104, 109

MCC. *See* Middle cingulate cortex (MCC)

MCS. *See* Motor cortex stimulation (MCS)

Medial prefrontal cortex
in rat model, 22–23

Medial thalamotomy (MT), 88–89

Mediodorsal thalamus, 104–106

MEG. *See* Magnetoencephalography (MEG)

Mesencephalotomy, 87–88

Middle cingulate cortex (MCC), 1

Midline myelotomy, 86

Migraine
and chronic tension-type headache, 24
sex-dependent structural/functional differences in, 34–35

Miniature inhibitory postsynaptic currents (mIPSCs), 108

MIPSCs. *See* Miniature inhibitory postsynaptic currents (mIPSCs)

Motor cortex stimulation (MCS), 79–81, 111–112

MRgFUS. *See* Magnetic resonance-guided focused ultrasound (MRgFUS)

MT. *See* Medial thalamotomy (MT)

Multivariate pattern analysis (MVPA), 129

MVPA. *See* Multivariate pattern analysis (MVPA)

Myelination, 21–22

N

Neocortex, 20, 132

Neurectomy, 82

Neuroablation, 82–90
anterolateral cordotomy (AC), 86–87
cingulotomy, 89–90
dorsal rhizotomy (DR), lesions, 83–84
dorsal root entry zone (DREZ) lesions, 83–84
dorsal root ganglionectomy (DRG), lesions, 83–84
facet blocks and denervations, 82
hypophysectomy, 85–86
medial thalamotomy (MT), 88–89
mesencephalotomy, 87–88
midline myelotomy, 86
neurectomy, 82
sympathectomy, 84–85

Neurogenesis, 19–20

Neuromodulation, 76–77, 133
by electricity, 133–136
by light, 136–138
by sound, 136
by visual cues, 138–139

Neuromodulation, 77–82
deep brain stimulation (DBS), 78–79
intrathecal opioids, 81–82
motor cortex stimulation (MCS), 79–81
peripheral nerve stimulation (PNS), 77
spinal cord stimulation (SCS), 77–78

Neuronal morphology/cerebral vasculature changes, 20

Neuroscientist, self-critique of, 139

Non-neuronal cell genesis and morphology, 20–21

Nurpin Pain Report, 8–9

O

OA. *See* Osteoarthritis (OA)

Opioid dependence effects, on brain structure and function, 33–34

Osteoarthritis (OA), 32
and gray matter changes in brain, 23*f*

Printed and bound by CPI Group (UK) Ltd, Croydon, CR0 4YY

03/10/2024

01040419-0010